TRAPPED

TRAPPED

My Life with Cerebral Palsy

FRAN MACILVEY

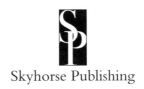

Skyhorse Publishing

I dedicate this book with deepest gratitude to my mother and father. With thanks to Dorothy Chitty, and Paul Lambillion, who showed me that dreams are worth believing and how to make them come true.

· · · · · · · · · · · · · · · · · ·

Author's Note

This narrative is an attempt to explain what living with a physical disability is like, for me and for those who have had the mixed fortune to live with me. Where I have had to imagine events or attribute motives or dialog, I have tried to be accurate and sympathetic. Where I have remembered circumstances, I have done my utmost to retell them as I believe they happened at the time. I hope that where I have taken liberties with the facts, this does not materially affect the narrative or cause offence. Errors in the text are mine alone.

· · · · · · · · · · · · · · · · ·

Chapter One

"Are you all right?"

This is my all-time favorite question, usually asked by concerned strangers with creased brows. Every time I fall, a flutter of enquiries greets me. Yet the chances are, if you are bending over to check whether I am all right, I have just tumbled hard to stony ground. Once again it has come up to meet me in a familiar, rough embrace, scraping skin off my knuckles or palms, which are now embedded with gravel, adding spots of blood to the muddy mess on my cuffs. Am I all right? I guess not, though I probably will be in a while.

It is good of you to ask and you are being very kind, but I am flat on my face. My spectacles are bent at a jaunty angle on my forehead, or are lying somewhere, glinting underfoot. Quickly, I grope for them before they get stepped on.

My daughter and I often traipse along the narrow canal pathway on the "school run," a welter of bikes, prams, dogs, and joggers whisking narrowly past. In the midst of wheels and staring schoolchildren, I make light of my body spread-eagled on the concreted towpath. I turn up my head and fix on a smile, the grin that suggests I am having the most marvelous time down here. If it is a quiet morning, I quip, "I am trying to get a tan!" or "I just fancied a rest," so that passers-by feel reassured. Once they are out of sight, I pull myself laboriously to my feet, sigh, and shuffle off again. Over and over this happens. I hate it, but have no choice.

I am not exceptional—only a middle-aged woman. I have almost forgotten that when I was younger I lived in Africa and ate home-harvested mangos, paw-paw, and passion fruit for breakfast. In the days before long-haul package holidays and well-meaning documentary makers crowding the game parks, we watched sentinel flamingos at dawn, yawning hippos stretching after a snooze, broad elephants placidly pulling breakfast from the ground nearby. We ate, slept, and lived in luxury, but not always happily.

Our family has had its share of problems, as all families do. But when I came along, everyday difficulties and disagreements skidded to the sidelines, while I and my problems dwelt unwillingly in the limelight; because I suffocated at birth, I have cerebral palsy, which makes walking in a calm, straight line impossible. My gait swings me from side to side. It is only with the helpful arm of a friend or an elbow crutch that my walking appears at all normal out of doors. Even then, I resemble an intransigent triangle, taking up more room than I should. In ultra-modern sneakers, I wobble like a drunkard, though other shoes are too uncomfortable to wear outside. As long as I have something to lean on, my wobblers help to straighten my back and take the strain off my knees and feet. They help me with the effort of walking.

"Excuse me!" puffs yet another sweaty jogger at my shoulder. I try to shrink myself further into the undergrowth, not because I aim, necessarily, to oblige; off the path, I stand less chance of being run down. By now I have sweat in my eyes and a stitch in my side, so I snatch a rest where no one will "'scuse me" for a few seconds.

My beloved daughter, her golden hair glinting in fresh spring sunlight, walks ahead and then waits patiently, wishing her daddy had brought her. When we start out in the streets around our apartment, it is all right for her to hold my hand. But the towpath is less roomy; and in any case, she doesn't want to be seen with me so much and would rather go by herself to school. Who could blame her? She walks with an easy, slim grace. I admire her strolling gentleness and wonder how such a calm, smooth creature could be my daughter. I, by contrast, sweat and inwardly swear, wishing I was anywhere but here.

Occasionally I ask myself whether I might prefer oblivion with its teasing mirage of soft comforts, but I have stopped saying, "I wish I had never been born" or "I wish I was dead" since these words do not help me to live a happy life. I used to run these phrases continuously in my head, before I understood how dangerous that is.

Welcome to my average day. All my days could be like this, especially when I forget to turn my tap of cheerfulness up to maximum. I must make a very deliberate effort not to cry, especially after I have fallen down somewhere public, busy, and humiliating. Landing untidily among nettles, plastic bags containing dog shit, potato chip bags, and half-empty beer cans is routine. I could write the definitive thesis on "How to Fall Safely" (most situations catered for). Even so, I regularly graze my hands and knees, or smear them with nameless messes that other people discard. I usually remember to take a hankie to help clean myself up. I cannot carry a faucet and towel with me. What would Seline say if I unbolted the kitchen sink and hauled it onto my back? "Come *on*, Mum, hurry up!"

On a good day I almost bounce. Once I fell head first down six deep stone steps at our local swimming pool and then got up and walked away, politely reassuring the astonished receptionist that I was unharmed. Though I felt like a circus performer, I make light of this talent simply because I have been falling since I first stood up. I am well into my forties, so the novelty of tumbling gracefully has worn off, replaced by a grim knowledge that I am no longer so good at mending. How long before I break a wrist, fracture a femur, or crack open my head? The question is beginning to feel old, as is the assorted patting, groping, and the sneers of the few folks who walk straight past me with their noses in the air. They must hear me muttering and decide that I am not right in the head. My bad temper is not aimed at them, but at falling yet again—I'm angry at *life!*

There are some who think I am a total disgrace to be collapsing drunk "at this time of day." Once, I pretended I had been drinking. I was a student—a young, smooth-faced girl with closely cropped hair, whom everyone mistook for a boy. On that morning I was walking home from the crowd of shabby stores on the main road, where you might find beer, discounted food, haphazard hardware: useful for a packet of fries or a jug of milk. I was going to get breakfast, when I tripped, flew, and—flump!—landed on the sidewalk. It was just my luck to have been seen by two well-intentioned habitués of the local bar, who assumed I had drunk too much amber nectar the night before and was just beginning to sober up. Before I knew what was happening, this pair of gentle gents hoisted me to my feet and, keeping their arms firmly under mine, decided to walk me home and make sure I could get the key in the lock of my front door. It wasn't far to go, just a block or two. They were joking so kindly, "Aye, lad, yev had a few too many last night, eh?" that I decided I would let them off. I didn't feel like being sniffy, hoity-toity, so I sank my voice as low as it would go, and carried on chatting in the local brogue, "Aye! O' righ'—Ah hiv 'n au! A wis stoopi' wis'n A'?!" Once they saw I had my key, they went away shaking their heads, pleased with theyselves for having bin so kind to this young man . . . shame he wis such a drinker, though.

When someone kind comes to help me, I believe in being as nice to them as possible. That can be a real challenge when I am sore, dirty, bleeding, embarrassed, and worried about my wrists. I have fallen hard on concrete perhaps fourteen thousand times. So, if you ever pick me up off the ground, please try to understand that any crossness that escapes from my well-controlled exterior, any apparent bad nature you may glimpse, has nothing whatsoever to do with you and everything to do with how I have to get by in this life.

Later, while my daughter is at school, I deal with a seemingly endless stream of household chores: washing, drying, cleaning, tidying, considering what we might have for supper. I ponder whether I must go out shopping. I have developed an intense dislike for the repetitions of domestic needs, yet I cannot seem to get away from them: carpets that need vacuuming, sheets to change, taps that leak, the plug that resists pulling and then slips from my fingers to roll uselessly on the floor.

The tasks to which I lend my attention feel pointless: endless petty patterns serving only to feed, wash, wipe, and mend. Feeling guilty for not being happily domestic, I hate hating it. But I have begun by inches to accept that small daily needs can serve, by their smallness, to mend a mind.

My mind is not broken—it never has been—yet my desires are so achingly wide and breathlessly high and my reach for them seems so futile, that sometimes only the basics can help, like making a cup of chicory coffee or starting another load of washing.

With an effort today to make a change of *something,* I choose a piece of music to keep me company, some of the Bach organ music I adore. Every time I hear this music, a picture of my father comes to mind, and I thank him fervently for making me sit and listen to these recordings when I was six years old. I have a date with Joh Seb Bach in heaven. When I meet this stout, wig-clad gentleman who speaks a clipped Thuringian German—which of course, I will understand perfectly—I will sit quietly beside him while he plays the spinet. I will tell him how much the music he left behind helped me to feel loved, to feel bliss and peace.

While throbbing, intimate threads of music build and recede like breathing, my mind flits uneasily to the past, wondering how to place on the page a reflection of my struggles, so that others can understand why it is that, despite my health, an apparently easy life running in straight lines without the complications of teenage pregnancy, divorce, or poverty, I still often wish I was someone else.

There are two women inside me. My first is the Fran who walks "in the public" and whom you think you understand. She is Seline's mom, who sorts her school bag and removes apple cores when they start to decompose, who cleans some of the clothes left lying around her bedroom floor. She is Eddie's wife, who dutifully turns up to school plays and parents' conferences (the thin, sloping head-teacher allows her considerable latitude in lateness for appointments).

This is the Fran who is met with smiles and "How are you?" and who has learned to answer dishonestly, for after all, some people have real hassle going on in their lives.

Should you look a little closer—though who among our friends looks really close?—you might notice what I don't talk about. With girlfriends I never mention sex, though I am happy to let them talk. Carefully, I allow them to overlook the fact that my contributions to conversations are not about me.

I know I am pretending. I pretend that I live a life like everybody else's. I pretend that my upbringing was straightforward; that my school days were filled with games, sports, girlish confidences, lipstick, love, and drama; that any time I want a job I can just go and get one; and that I have a sex life that is fairly normal.

By pretending, I gift myself the appearance of a normal life, and I begin to believe that a normal life is what I have achieved. So part of me feels good, happy, ordinary. The rest is often angry, antisocial, and unhappy. Anger comes in surges, sweeping painfully through my head, throbbing behind my eyes. I have an energy that flares dangerously, or lies limp and lost, like a pile of gray ash, exhausted.

Perhaps one day, standing beneath the unfurling crown of a vast tree in the rain, I may become friends with the water pelting across my shoulders. I might even melt and vanish. For a bright second or two, this bone-tired body would be weightless, and I would feel myself soaring.

Chapter Two

A deep breath, and it all begins. A deep sigh, some loving impregnation, and *voila*! I am on my way. The healers and angel talkers I consult later say, "Your soul made a choice to come into this world as you did." Some of the books I have read mention karmic debts, wheels and roundabouts, cause and effect. These answers strike chords within, and in my dreams, I get some replies to anguished questions: vivid colored slates of meaning sent for me to read; shapes and puns. So now I can almost accept. On waking each morning, remnants of the old sorrow stir uneasily in my chest. Unless I push them firmly to one side, ancient voices may come creeping, repeating, "Why me?"

I am a mere slip of a girl, a forty-something mother, yet each dawning day feels etched into my skin, and my sorrow for all the times when I have lived less than gently with myself and less than happily, pushes down over my shoulders. My face appears youthfully misleading, framed with abundant dark hair trying to lift into curls. I have fair skin and a smile that charms anyone who comes up close, until I fall or stagger awkwardly. No one seems to want to hang too near after that, in case my bumps and the few glimpses of caress I venture turn to clutching, revealing deeper needs.

How does anything start? Nobody is perfect. I am Fran, born on the second of January, a stupid birth date that Mum often overlooked. Each turn of the year the question would surface, "What on earth have I forgotten?" and rest uncomfortably between her shoulder blades. "Oh, for God's sake! The twins' birthday!" And on the fourth or thereabouts, when we had regained some enthusiasm for parties, there would be presents rescued from around the house and wrapped afresh. My mother is a genius at improvisation. I make light of this fate, the chance that gave my sister and me as a New Year's present to a woman who already had two children under four years old.

Mum has not spoken to me directly about the night before I was born. Like many of her contemporaries, she does not talk openly of what has gone before, but rather in apologetic snatches when she thinks no one is listening. My father will not speak of things long past. He must think, by now, that I know.

So perhaps they will excuse me if I *ad lib* and suggest that my mother would have been feeling tired after celebrating Christmas with the time-honored formality of most well-heeled Europeans living in the tropics: endless, rather pointless parties fuelled by locally brewed alcohol or an unreliable supply of imported gin. Crates of soft drinks found at the local markets were a particular help, as anything not obtained nearby had to be freighted in from Europe—medicines, alcohol, candles, matches, clothes, and food—and a container of goods could take many months to arrive, transported first by sea to the west coast of Africa and then up the wide Congo River to Kinshasa. Even so, hot on the heels of Santa and his reindeer, yesterday's New Year blowout fell on a Friday, offering a perfect excuse for yet another "do," the night before my sister and I made our appearance.

In the golden glow of dozens of lights strung artfully under the eaves of the terrace, strangers would have been lounging, their faces dimly lit—assuming the generator was working. When the power failed, flickering candles lit the pathways.

Raucous celebrations disguised a constant fear: The Belgian Congo during the 1960s was a powder keg of intrigue and clandestine assassinations. Reckless alliances were hatched among careless guests and visitors who spent evenings hovering anxiously on the fringes of parties or getting drunk poolside. The hostess of this party would rather have been taking a well-earned rest in a cool bath, alone and peaceful.

Having left school at the top of her class, Estelle pursued medical studies with distinction before giving them up to marry Kristof. It seemed very romantic at the time, but on discovering that her husband, newly recruited to the Belgian diplomatic corps, was being sent to the Congo, she wept: If a white man had any desire to die young, a posting there in the midst of a simmering rebellion would shorten his odds considerably; and if he was Belgian, to write his will before he set off was sensible, no matter his age.

But against the odds, Kristof Freyerling and his wife put down shy roots in the deep, welcoming African soil. And despite their northern habits, the seductive brooding power of Africa cast its spell over them.

Beyond the warm cocoon of flickering lights, in the deep shadows of night, frogs and toads croaked by the pool. Dogs howled at the moon, while in the humming darkness, tree dwellers crept on silent tiptoe among swaying branches. In this vast continent of dripping tropical forests, surging rivers, and blazing skies, nights are deep velvet blue, richly scented with the sweet fragrances of wide open flowers wilting softly, their scents enticing a sonorous assortment of winged visitors.

In the enfolding darkness, a man from the forest with exceptionally sharp hearing and a long knife stood, on orders to keep watch over the house and grounds. While all around stories of robbery and death were whispered, our family was kept safe; they said the night watchman had special powers. Less mystically, Mum carried a loaded handgun in her car, which she wasn't afraid to use against hijackers. Word got around that we should be left alone.

On the stone balconies, loud guests sang tunelessly, belched and hugged each other, nursing hangovers from yesterday's party. These people inhabited a rarefied world of canapés and cracked crab. Missing the refinements of home, they nibbled like scavengers at tilted plates of strewn food, longed for a warm Belgian beer, and politely agreed that the provisions were excellent.

Sinuous Congolese jazz spun in a lopsided dance with patriotic but tuneless military marches. Too much enjoyment of local musical brilliance would have been frowned upon, so my father alternated the tracks—one lovely, the next laughable—and everyone was happy. The reel-to-reel tape deck was perched precariously on the veranda, hooked up to a loudspeaker atop the flagpole in the garden. Servants passed by in their smart white evening jackets edged with gold trim. They wore immaculate white gloves. The guests were free to leer, belch, and paw other men's wives; but black hands must never touch the food.

Expecting her third child, this evening Estelle glowed self-consciously, the festive mood slipping past her. As sweat trickled gently down between her shoulders and prickles of discomfort shimmied up her spine, she reminded herself sternly that her baby was not due tonight. Standing five feet four inches in gold sandals, Estelle endured sly winks and nudges, "Big Mama! Big boy!" Six weeks to go.

"Well, *Madame* Freeling, how about a nightcap to see in the New Year, eh?" Estelle fixed on her bright smile and was considering her reply when there was a sharp kick in her abdomen, and a new layer of cold sweat broke over her neck. Voices sounded hollow, faces swam out of focus, and there was a taste like metal in Estelle's mouth. She muttered, "Beg your pardon, sorry . . ." and tottered away in search of Kristof. Hostess service temporarily suspended.

In a fluttering panic, Estelle moved through the crowd, her eyes searching. "Celestine? Look after the children, please? I must go."

"*Oui, Madame*, of course."

A thin, dark man, his face carefully blank, sidled past carrying a tray of dirty glasses shoulder high. Estelle asked, "Have you seen *Monsieur*?" He nodded slightly, with a small movement of his head indicating that her husband could be found in the study downstairs. My mother staggered as calmly as she could over the wooden flooring. Heaving the door ajar, she hovered, aware of different weights bearing down on her: the dark doorframe, her swollen stomach, her anxious heaviness, so unlike a hostess should be. A heaving pulse pressed, and Estelle swallowed.

"Daudi!" Father called out to the night watchman. "Daudi!" Feet scampered to attention and gates were inched open. Servants stood in the flicker of generated lights as the "Land Rover" was driven from the garage. Everything seemed to move slowly, heavy in the muggy heat. In his haste, Kristof called out unnecessarily, "I am going—*C'est Madame—Ma femme!*" Opening the passenger door, Kristof helped his wife up into her seat. As she lifted her legs, there was a small flood over the seat, drenching her sandals.

Chapter Three

Two young white people skirting dirt paths and moving hastily along the corridors of the newly opened hospital at night attracted curious stares. The facility was open, though sleepy. Queues of African women, children, and old men lined the hallways or lolled on the veranda, waiting their turn with the medical men in the morning. Meanwhile, quiet murmurs and whispered coughs filled the air. Cigarette smoke floated above dim light, as hands reached out to help Estelle. She was hoisted competently and quickly onto a couch, and at the last moment she remembered to ask Kristof to stay.

"Stay?" The senior doctor on duty that night was a shabby, balding man wearing stained overalls. He grimaced, a sneer of doubt pursing his lips. "You would like to stay? *Eh bien*, it is most irregular, *Monsieur*, but if you insist . . ." It was obvious that an extra body would be a hindrance in the cramped space around the bed. Yet, with quiet defiance, Kristof placed his wife's wrist under his arm in a gentle, protective gesture. In this hospital, among strangers, they held hands. As Estelle's life swam out of focus, there was only his clasp, and unknown voices, urging her to breathe, to wait, to push. It continued for minutes, or hours, time meant nothing. The pain was always the same.

As the first yellow and orange tinges lit up a dark blue sky of dawn, small screams pulsed from the stretching, wretched woman lying prone on the couch. Smeared with sweat and blood, Estelle was exhausted and sore. Useless nurses crowded around her, ignoring her shyness and careless for her modesty—their endless chattering! She wished her mother—oh, God!—she wished her mother were here.

The prayerful vigil of the young parents was abruptly splintered, brusquely broken up by the senior surgeon pushing through bodies in his way. "So here we are then, heh? And not long now, *Madame!*" This man, supposedly in charge, wielded a slippery bravura that hinted at boozing on the sly, this weekend of the New Year.

"Gently, now . . . and now, push!" Meekly, Estelle obeyed though she was exhausted, her body spinning with sharp agonies. "Eh, bravo! See *Madame*, a beautiful baby!" The surgeon grinned as the midwife held aloft a very small, very quiet child, a girl. She was suspended, hung at a distance and slapped so that she cried out in her first anger, her first sorrow.

"You have done well, see!" The words were brave, although uncertainty hovered: this baby was not big. Fresh out of her mother's womb, the child was weighed, tagged, and measured, while Estelle looked on helplessly. Presently, her baby's tiny, bundled body was returned to her side and placed in her arms while Kristof looked on, dazed by new beauty. It all seemed unreal, as it does when you gain a child; now they noticed that doctors were explaining patiently, the baby was too tiny, she must go immediately to the incubators and *Madame* should rest. Everything would be attended to.

Estelle swallowed back tears and lay obedient and still.

In a loud voice an attendant was saying, "And the father can please leave?" At the prospect of losing him, Estelle jolted into wakefulness, her face creased in fretful lines. "Small?" she whispered.

Kristof nodded.

"But, how? That cannot be! She must be at least five pounds!"

"No, much less."

"Then why . . .?" Her question died on her lips, as she was seized by another familiar pulse, terrifying. Impossible.

Voices were repeating, "*Madame* must rest now!"

Estelle cried, "No, Kristof! Stay . . . please stay . . .?" Her husband shrugged narrow shoulders as Estelle was seized by an overwhelming urge to push. She winced, her words jolting in a thread of disbelief, "For God's sake; there is another one coming! Help me, please!"

Kristof came to her side, nodded, and ran off to find anyone who would listen. There was no one. Ten minutes passed. All the staff was busy, in no doubt that his proper place was outside in the hallway: no patience for him. Twenty minutes passed. He darted from bed to bed, trying to summon into his slim, boyish body sufficient authority to command a hearing. Hands waved him aside. Why would he not go, go and rest in the corridor, out of the way?

Time ticked on: thirty minutes.

"She needs help, don't you understand?"

At last the consultant lent his ear to the hopping noise at his side.

"My wife is having another baby."

"What do you say?"

"My—wife has another—baby on the way! Quick! Come quickly!"

The man in charge turned and looked down at the groveling youth. Years of training had taught him well, how to be conciliatory and dismissive at the same time. "*Monsieur* Freyerling, I am the doctor here, heh? And you, you are the . . . euh . . . consul. I let you do your job? And of course, you will let me do mine! *Naturellement!* You have a child, a beautiful child. And we are doing our very best for her right now. What more do you want?" The older man moved away, rudely shouldering past. Forty minutes.

"I will show you, if you don't believe me!" Father was shouting now, frantic, his voice precisely the breaking, boyish plea most likely to be ignored. He ran to rejoin Estelle, still laboring alone in her bed, where everyone thought she was sleeping. At her side, Kristof placed his hands over her stomach in a gesture of tenderness and entreaty. Quickly his right hand sought her vulva, finding an unmistakable hardness of sinew.

Someone would have followed, to ensure that this lunatic my father didn't cause any more disturbance. Now Dad's shadow was gesturing frantic hand signals behind his back to assemble a crowd of helpers. "You see?" The top man again muscled in, looked down and for once was too shocked to say anything, except, "Ah, my God, what have we here?" These immortal words greeted my entry into planet earth.

Fifty-five minutes late, there now, between his hands slid into the world a child with a grossly swollen head, a blue body wrapped in yards of cord.

Wrapped in knots of sorrow and fury, I was a crumpled, ugly bundle. My head was bloated, my limbs somehow tacked on; yards of cord pulled around my neck cutting off air, slicing my body—and strength—in two. I was trapped.

A nurse said quickly, with forced conviction, swallowing most of her words in panic, "See, here is another daughter for you!" She spoke bravely into dislocated silence. From the bodies near her, my mother heard, "the umbilicus . . ." and understood all the rest.

Estelle's tears fell. It would have been all right, she was thinking, if only someone had listened. "My child!" she murmured. "Poor child!" Clinging to the wrapped bundle for a few precious seconds, she entreated that her strength would do for us both. From somewhere deep within, bubbles of sadness and joy rose together—twins! Girls! The last thing anyone suspected.

By now Mum was exhausted, unable to stop her newest daughter being pried firmly from her and carried away for special care alongside her sister. Delivery into the hands of others. At six weeks premature, we were too small for comfort. No one knew whether death would come for either of us.

As the rest of the hospital was coming to life and Mum fell into jerky sleep, Father took his chance to slip away. Exhausted, he sat numbly on the porch smoking a calming cigarette while he pondered the twist of fate that had delivered two new, fragile daughters into his care. He had expected to feel elation and pride, not this sorrow he could not shift from his throat; anguish made worse by a soft hum of pity following at his back. No one met his eyes. No one smiled widely. Should one say, "Congratulations," which might sound a little unkind?

My sister was and still is a limpid beauty, with piercing blue-gray eyes like her father's and a gentle, giving temperament. Together, we were incubated at the hospital while Estelle looked on. During our first day of life outside the womb, my father asked for the priest, a quiet man who nodded gravely and murmured words of hasty baptism and the last rites over us in his heavily accented Latin, all of which drove Estelle into a frenzy of grief.

During long, solitary nights surrounded by shadows crawling to daybreak and filled with fear, our mother simply had to pull herself together. She had to keep us all going. At her insistence, her girls were brought from the nursery every hour to be fed. Getting us latched on while we were tiny was impossible. Hovering nurses, bringing their unwelcome mixture of condolences and old wives' tales, began to mutter about formula milk, but Estelle was abruptly dismissive: In a place where there was no guarantee with the water supply, what did they know? She persevered with a heavy glass breast pump that slipped clumsily in her hands. Her milk was collected and fed to us using droppers. Jars fell and smashed on the floor. Mother wept, heavy with frustration and mourning. She forced herself to eat, to sleep, while a suffocating depression waited at every corner.

Visitors mumbled that our chances were slim and left, shaking their heads. This was Africa, after all, a primitive backwater. Yet, as each new day dawned, my sister and I clung lightly to life. Lying side by side we snoozed happily and gained weight.

One afternoon, my parents arranged for us to be properly christened Martha Laura and Frances Mary, and there was a subdued celebration. The following day, it was agreed we could leave the glass incubator.

Martha Laura kept her angelic sweetness and generosity of temperament. Accepting everything, she gazed placidly about her as her days passed by. I was different: cross and mottled, crumpled and angry. My limbs did not lie in smooth lines.

Chapter Four

On the last day of January, our discharge papers were signed off and left aside for Mum to collect from the main office at the hospital. She and the consultant exchanged words about me, though it was years before I learned what was discussed.

The young *ayah* Celestine, who had been taken on to care for the children of our household, was herself a girl of sixteen, with three brothers and two sisters of her own. Celestine was the European name her family gave her, wrapping it snugly among her more familiar African ones. As yet, no one in her employer's household could speak Lingala well, though Father, a natural linguist, was improving quickly.

The afternoon Mum came home from the hospital with Martha and me, Celestine had my brother clasped on her hip; he was pulling her braids gently and fingering shiny glass beads of blue, white, yellow, and red that were threaded around her throat. Simon was the *ayah*'s little pet. He had a sweet, round face with hooded eyes. Quiet, intelligent, and serious, he listened while she spoke, laughingly joined in her singing as she worked, clapping his hands and thumping his legs as she danced. He played happily in the sun, a floppy bleached hat perched on his head.

His older sister had taken herself off somewhere. She enjoyed exploring. She was unlikely to be alone: in Africa no white girl is solitary for long. Elouise greatly enjoyed playing under bushes with any nearby child, pet, or insect. In her secret life away from her parents, she smiled and danced playfully, free from the usual expectations of good behavior.

Elouise was very beautiful, with angelic features framed by bleached blond curls. Where her brother was peaceful, quiet, and gentle, Elouise was voluble, demanding, and demonstrative. She adored parties, people, and games of all sorts. Between them, this girl and her younger brother had grown up a truce, so that they could share their parents' attention in relative peace. Until now, there had been space for them both, since their temperaments were so different, but everything changed after Martha and I came home.

Celestine was out in the dusty backyard pulling together dried laundry. Shifting noises at the front of the house marked the return home: gates juddering open, a tone of voice that answered shortly, a breeze of unfamiliar formality. As the least important member of this household, she did not rush out to the front driveway. She walked placidly to find Elouise, who was preoccupied with making a skirt of leaves for one of her dolls. In the dust, her face was smeared as if she had been eating ants. Quickly wiping the child's face with the palm of her free hand, the *ayah* grasped Elouise's wrist and walked calmly to the front of the house to wait. It was all over the district, the news that *Madame* had twin daughters, and that one of them was damaged—ayee! Twins were a great honor, a sign of heavenly blessing and masculine fertility, but it was boys who were especially desired. Uncertainty hovered over a baby girl with a twisted body.

Chapter Five

"Mum?" There was a long, scratchy pause on the line Estelle had booked to speak to her parents. At three pounds for three minutes, this tenuous gap in space was not cheap.

"Yes, Estelle dear, I'm here."

"It's good that you and Dad are coming to see us, Mum, you can catch up with the children." Estelle weighed her words carefully. "How much progress Fran is making these days! She can lift her head up now and pulls herself everywhere with her arms."

"What about the others?"

Estelle felt a spasm of frustration: her mother was saying she must not neglect the rest of her family. From long habit, she forced a smile into her voice. "They are fine, Mum, having lots of fun. I will come and get you from the airport. Just wait for me."

Ten days later, my mother stood in a small room called "Arrivals" waiting for her parents to make it through customs. There were fewer formalities than usual, perhaps because Stuart and Eleanor looked so obviously like tourists, rather awkwardly clutching a suitcase each and sweating in the bright heat. They looked startled, as if the brightness hurt their eyes.

Plain words of greeting sounded strange, at odds with the generous confusion that surrounded them. Though she hugged her mother warmly and kissed her father affectionately on both cheeks, Estelle would find it hard to relax until everything had been explained and found to be acceptable to her parents. They had travelled a long way to be with her.

Simon and Elouise were playing outside in the garden with Martha. Sounds of laughter and quarrelling drifted lazily around the house. As usual, the afternoon was warm and bright, with high clouds soaring, blown gently in vivid blue heavens. The men of the house, Grandpa Stewart and Father, chatted companionably on the veranda, cradling post-prandial drinks while their women, Grandma Eleanor and Estelle, were busy indoors. Both women were sitting back on their heels, watching me.

"Would you like to see what she can do?" My mother had pulled off my top and placed me on a mat between them. I rolled over onto my front, and smilingly pushed my tummy up off the floor with a grunt of effort. I was pink and puffing, but Mum saw unmistakable pride in me pushing down my hands. There was determination and freedom there; I was going for a medal.

Gently, treading carefully, Eleanor asked, "Is that all? A baby of two-and-a-half should be managing . . . more?"

Mummy huffed in exasperation. "She is getting better every day! She holds up her head now. We give her massages, movement, support. I have lots of help with this. You can see how much happier Fran is."

"Well," said Eleanor, who was only thirty-six hours into her month-long stay with her daughter's family, "I wouldn't know about that, but I'll take your word for it."

Stung to disappointment, Estelle bit back her tears. "I thought you would be more pleased."

"I am, dear, it is just that she is so slow, don't you think? Is all your work making a difference, or are you just chasing a dream and neglecting the others? What does Kristof say about all this time you spend on Fran?"

"I know the others don't get enough of my attention but how can I dole out my time fairly? At least they can play with each other. And Fran is getting better every day. Should I just give up and let her take her chances? As far as I can tell, she might end up in a wheelchair if I abandon her now. Is that what you want?"

"Of course not" Eleanor soothed. "It just doesn't seem fair to the rest of the family, that's all."

The women gazed blankly into the middle distance, perhaps trying to see what the future held. In the silence, I pushed myself up and for the first time, caught my leg underneath my stomach and made a move to crawl forward. Neither woman noticed, though on my face there was an even bigger smile than usual.

Chapter Six

Little children patter happily about, peering at stockings, puzzling at shoes, buckles, and laces. I watched and felt excitement in tiny details: my mother's elegant leather sandals lined up on the bottom of her wardrobe; the shimmering fabric of her bright dresses patterned a dazzling array of oranges and reds. Down the large stairway, crawling under armchairs, I peeled back rugs, tilting my head at odd sounds and strange company. The music that Father chose for us to listen to was filled with thrilling tunes that made me dance, laughing and spinning in clumsy pirouettes, or galloping round the border of the afghan carpet pretending to be a lion or a cheetah. After the excitement, once I had calmed down, I looked out for the tom cat that lived with us in his own strictly part-time arrangement. Whisky was a thin streak of black; a greedy, solitary beast who rarely tolerated affectionate petting. When food was out, he was in, eating all he could. The rest of the time, the creature kept to himself, only seen occasionally streaking wildly over the floors of the house in the evenings, his eyes on the bats and mice that lurked tantalizingly out of reach up in the curtains. I crawled while my siblings ran, so it was often forgotten that I could understand far more than any "normal" crawling child would.

I saw them looking at me. I thought they were waving, so I pulled myself along—so fast—to go and see. To get up, I tugged table cloths, pulled the backs of chairs, and leaned heavily. There were many smiles and pats on the head. There were other whisperings too, enquiring glances, voices hushed or hard. Murmurs and smirks when I slid, rolled, and fell.

When I was almost three years old, I sat upright and promptly slipped sidey-ways under the table. How funny to watch! The family laughed and I was merry. I sloped sideways and quietly slid to the floor. But then how annoying it became to retrieve me from the house dogs and the fluff on the floor. Father was puzzled, irritated at my evident lack of progress. The laughter started again, and later the frowns.

Chapter Seven

Aged three, I recall the thrill of being aboard an enormous ship with my mother. She tells me that I once got tipsy on sips of whisky offered by genial gentlemen taking their first tipple of the morning. A clutch of elderly ladies enjoying a stroll on deck said smilingly, "Isn't she lively this morning!" mistaking my drunken somersaults for high spirits. I remember the delight of ringing the bell for dinner; my mother dressing in elegant clothes to go out, leaving me in the cabin. I could not work out what the shadowy sailor clambering around outside and throwing ropes was doing. I hoped he was not a robber.

It never occurred to me to wonder what would happen to Martha, Simon, and Elouise while we were away travelling, in all likelihood to meet orthopedic experts and consultants in London. With typical childish egocentricity, I didn't give it much thought. In our absence, they formed alliances that would later tend to exclude me: I was the lucky one who was going on adventures, while they were abandoned, sent to stay with a cruel and neglectful neighbor for the several weeks that they were left behind at home.

Perhaps to make amends, on our return we all—barring Father, the servants, or the cook—decamped for the holiday of a lifetime to Mombasa, the port of Kenya.

Aged three and a half, I sat watching wind-puffed sand beetles and waves. I looked on as my amazing mummy erected a vast canvas tent for us all to sleep under. The smell of the oiled cloth, the zip of the tent flap, the potty for pissing in: all these I loved. Mum set up a calor gas stove out front, where we ate with an exhilarating lack of rules, happily scoffing food from tins and packets. Everything else was cooked on the two rings of camping gas or roasted over a cracking wood fire.

I looked up at high palms nestling hard-shelled coconuts that were cut down, sliced open with a sharp *panga* knife, and offered to us. Clumsily, I drank the sweet juice, which ran over my chin and dripped onto the sand. Left in peace to sit and watch the waves, my fingers found fun digging out shells, popping heads of seaweed, and gouging deep holes to tumble into. Wearing thin gym shoes, I splashed in rock pools, safe from the cutting coral lurking in the shallow water.

I had my first encounter with true love, brought to me by an elderly auntie who raised me up from my usual crawl and embraced me. She took me leaping into waves breaking on the shore. Holding each other upright, we jumped, me gazing into her smiling face and being lifted up. "Here it comes . . . wait for it . . . WHOOSH!" We giggled and shrieked, this woman and I, in the age-old conspiracy of the elderly with infants. It was the first of several infatuations with women who were not my mother.

That holiday also brought its share of pain and irritation, when I got my third of a dozen sets of stitches in an encounter with a rock. My knee thought it was stronger and got badly cut. Blood flowed, salting the water along with my tears. Mummy and the *ayah* scooped me up and a hospital visit was hastily organized: I remember iodine and plasters, sorry words, and consoling hugs.

I also recall Mum chasing me over sand, brandishing a tube of eye drops. I fought like a wild cat until she could no longer be bothered to overcome my resistance to her good intentions. I breathed a sigh of relief as, with a few cross words, she surrendered the pursuit and finally left me to myself.

That holiday marked a small watershed. It was the beginning of all my happiest memories. During that time at the beach, it also began to filter into my awareness that I was the child who had things "done" to her, a sort of ongoing experiment or improvement project. "Getting Better" my father called it. Push and shove, and with a sigh of magic, all would be fixed. The only question was: where to start?

At the age of six months, I am told, I had improvement surgery for my eyelids, after which I would have been confined to a hospital bed. I am grateful every time I look in a mirror, although I seem to have been left with a phobia for curved iron bedsteads painted white, which sparks a rising nausea. The unusual shape of my eyelids remains a source of comment; healthy teeth have been extracted and the remainder straightened; I have been forced to wear ugly, uncomfortable shoes; my feet have been mutilated; and I have been stretched on couches and examined more often than any child should have to endure. To further the cause of medical science—not for my benefit—I have even been filmed.

As a shy late developer of fifteen, all I knew was that I walked rather like a monkey and had difficulty getting in and out of the bath. However, according to the physiotherapists at my local orthopedic hospital, the cerebral palsy I have is a most unusual variety, a rare inversion of the more obvious oddities one might expect to see. It was explained to my mother and me that the doctors wanted permission to use my "case" for studies with their medical students. "Would you mind?" I was asked, though no one supposed I might answer back, "Yes, I would mind very much, actually." My mother, familiar with the needs of clinical research, agreed easily, so who was I to object?

On the appointed day, behind a screen in a large shabby hall, surrounded by gawking medical staff and junior doctors anxious to impress one another, I undressed down to my underpants and put on a swimming costume that a physiotherapist had found for me in a box of odds and ends. Then I walked for them all. They watched closely, taking notes and peering at me, as, solitary in my oddness, I paraded up and down a strip of dusty red carpet, the physiotherapist directing my pathway so that I could be viewed to best advantage. The cine camera whirred away in the background. The operator wanted to get the angles just right. He moved this way and that, peering to see everything, "very grateful." After much discussion, stretching, and calibration, I was allowed to get dressed.

Chapter Eight

When we were very young, we lived in a home that stood in discreetly wooded acres, nestled amidst the hills above Nairobi. In the grounds below the house there was a tennis court and a swimming pool where we spent most of our free time. In between, great banks of flowers towered above us like scented waterfalls. Bougainvillea bushes played host to fragile butterflies and harmless lizards. We gazed up in wonder at the shadowy haunts of humming bees.

The magical home we borrowed for two years has, like its neighbors, long since been bulldozed to make way for crowded blocks of apartments, housing the families of people who actually live locally, which is just as well: the locals were forever standing at a respectful distance outside the gates. As I grew older and more aware of the disparities in our lives, I became uncomfortable with the deference and privileges I enjoyed. I would rather have been running and playing as the local children did, who gnawed on maize cobs and sugar cane.

Because of Father's employment, every two or three years we flitted, and our next move was to the shore of the Indian Ocean on the coast of Tanzania. The residence we then occupied sat proudly on the main road directly opposite the beach so that our whole days were modulated by the sounds of waves. While Elouise, Simon, and Martha pelted round the house and grounds, skipping and laughing, I propped myself against the wall at the kitchen step. My legs were not holding me up, so I didn't join in much. Not yet, though I usually found company near the house: during long, hot days, a cool space in the shade was precious. The family dogs delighted in lying over my lap, their heads lolling in the afternoon heat. I stroked their soft muzzles and swore I would never leave them.

From afar, I adored the brother who was forever playing tricks on me.

"Fran, see that plane over there?" Simon would challenge, knowing that I couldn't resist a bet.

Looking up into the sky I would see a moving dot, and nod.

"Well, if it is coming in to land, I will give you a shilling, and if it is taking off, you will give me one, okay?" "Yeah, okay . . ." and I would hand over a shilling a couple of minutes after we had both watched the plane rise up and soar away into the distance.

The house staff working about the kitchens observed me seated solitarily on the kitchen step and tutted with regret. They passed me dishtowels wrapped around tarnished silver for my fingers to polish as I listened happily to their relaxed conversations and laughter. I enjoyed watching Mr. Adams, the cook, as he deftly moved about issuing gentle instructions to the houseboy, or spent the morning whipping egg whites with a small, bent fork to make soufflé.

To my eyes, the kitchen was small and sparsely furnished, with few of the modern conveniences we take for granted. Yet Mr. Adams' puddings—especially his chocolate soufflé, strawberry tart, and angelica ice cream—were among the best I have tasted.

I often returned to that bright perch at the back door, from where I could look out on the world, watching movement. There was much to see in the wide open spaces. I learned that it was exciting to listen to silence: I waited for the flick of rain on parched red earth under a brooding storm, for far-off claps of thunder coming closer and fizzing flashes that flared pink, yellow, and silver. As thunder rolled and the rain drenched, I laughed. God seemed to say, "Little girl, see! My red earth is filled with life; my beasts that soar, crawl, and run through bushes, up trees, and across the wide plains."

While we played as we liked, our parents living so far from their paler northern homes had a great deal to do simply to keep us healthy and properly fed. Malaria, waterborne diseases, and deadly fevers, snake bites, termites, jellyfish, mosquitoes, and cockroaches all added to the challenges of normal child rearing, yet none of us children was ever seriously ill.

Mummy caught black water fever once, and in the grip of deathly weakness, drove herself to the hospital for drug treatments that saved her life. But she does not talk about that episode. As always, with a touching faith that things would come out right if she worked hard enough at them, she got on with what she had to do.

To contrive sufficient food to eat was an ongoing battle, and our food stores were constantly pilfered from the cold room, a situation which was largely tolerated. The servants were allowed to take food, cigarettes, and alcohol as part of their wages, though Father rather sternly questioned anyone asking for a half bottle of scotch. He did not want his staff turning up drunk for work.

Despite the appearance of leisure, much time was spent in thankless experiments with food. Thus, Mum acquired two pairs of rabbits and set about breeding them for meat. Mr. Adams and the houseboy thought nothing of dispatching them for the pot and there was much laughter and games of catch when they escaped through the wire fencing. Rabbits abound! Before six months passed, we had dozens of fluffy hoppers cooped up round the house: rabbit stew, rabbit fricassee, rabbit curry with mango, roast rabbit with corn fritters, roast rabbit and cassava bake. After nine months we had eaten enough sweet, gamey flesh from those docile creatures never to want it again. As quickly as they came to dominate the table, they disappeared, the only reminders of their existence a few wisps of fluff clinging to the barbs in the fence. After that, it was fish.

Later still, in quiet testimony to Father's advancement in the service, tinned luxuries like ravioli and asparagus, cornflakes imported at great expense, and apples shipped from Europe appeared regularly at the table. I loved the smell of the apples, which came in large boxes, snuggly packed on the blue polystyrene trays, which are still used in packaging to this day. Boisterous and ungrateful like children everywhere, we took most of these efforts for granted.

Clothing was less of a problem. We happily slummed around the house wearing an assortment of much used cut-downs and bare feet. Every so often Mum would put out a clarion call, "Right, children, get dressed, I am taking photos to send to Grandma and Grandpa!" Despite the heat, we reluctantly pulled on our smartest clothes—with socks as well as shoes—otherwise there would have been complaints. "Goodness, Estelle, the children look so dreadfully *scruffy,* don't they?"

Chapter Nine

After breakfast, on a morning much like any other, I sloped upstairs to wash. The cool bathroom at the back of the house, home to small, grateful geckos sheltering from the heat, had a toilet with an old-fashioned high cistern that gurgled affectionately when the chain was pulled. It was my habit not to lock the door as the catch was heavy and difficult, and I didn't want to get stuck. When I shimmied off the seat, splashed water on my hands and face, and moved across the floor, the door would not open. No matter how I pulled, the unyielding metal lock did not budge. I called to be let out, but no one heard or came to see. It was a big house in which sounds just floated away.

I sat on the floor. Time passed while I played. I looked at the ceiling and contemplated the wallpaper, until there was a grating sound as Father turned the key in the lock and lifted me away. I was thinking there must have been a mistake until it dawned on me that the rest of the family had been over the road to the beach, and Elouise admitted crossly she did not want me there getting in the way. She apologized, with a little persuasion from our frowning father. The starkness of her resentment—whap!—hit me like a slap. It was such a small thing, yet the realization that my siblings rejoiced in their freedom *without me* sent a shaft of pain through me that gripped, shook, and refused to let go.

That morning, I understood clearly that when others looked at me, they saw a nuisance. It was my first taste of the loneliness that would come to dominate.

My copious tears were wept and swept aside. "Come now, Fran, what is there to cry about?" My smile would come back. I was just me, happy because the world unfolding around me was so beautiful. Many hugs and kisses were mine. I had piggyback rides, swept up in a beach towel on Father's back. I was watched carefully and with much love, though I was contrary and often difficult to please: Did I want helping with this thing, or that? No, I usually liked to manage by myself. Did I need help? Yes, sometimes I did, though I was not often appreciative. It must have been difficult and frustrating for the family to be on hand, forever unsure which help I would enjoy and what I would resent and remember forever.

I had been taught that it was polite to listen when others were speaking, though my position as the youngest meant that my words were not often heard. Opinions about me seemed to be traded freely while I was expected to nod politely, rarely to contribute. I often felt uncomfortable. Yet, when I asked questions or wanted to know where my confusion and anger were coming from, my desire to please choked off most of my frustration. Anyway, perhaps I would fit in more easily if I was silent and spoke up for myself less often . . .

As a regretful scold, "You are very lucky!" was offered to my sullen face. These words gave me no comfort in my rages of frustration or sorrow, instead adding guilt to the mix. I nodded without understanding, or simply got crosser. It was never going to be easy to answer my questions. Why was I "lucky" to be unhappy? Should I be filled with joy, with legs like sticks that left me marooned on the kitchen step or at the beach, while the rest of my handsome, mobile family played games, danced, swam, or went snorkeling and diving?

My mother noticed the endless balancing act that left me tongue-tied. She saw clouds over my eyes that spoke of my unhappiness. Wisely, she handed me crayons and gave me lines to draw; or she took me upstairs and cut my hair to soothe me. With her, I was often allowed to cry and let go of my sorrow.

Too young to explain how I felt, I often took revenge for my frustration on those who would be most forgiving and least likely to hold me to account for my unkindness. Martha gave me time and attention that I scarcely deserved. When she would have been happier doing other things, I wheedled, "Make my bed for me, wait for me, help me," though I was perfectly capable of managing most daily routines, and in any case, we had servants to do the housework. She yielded continuously to my demands and I wasn't even thankful.

I remember once at the beach, I threw a heavy stick at Martha; it hit her on the side of the face so that her nose bled and she had to be carried home, but I was not sorry. Another afternoon, she cycled out alone to the local swings, in a play area called "The Green." She knew she was not allowed beyond the gates by herself, and I was upset that she had gone away and left me, whizzing off with such glee. When, driving home, Mum spotted her familiar shape on the main road, she chased her back to the house. Reaching the bedroom in record time, Martha panted, "Don't tell Mum!" as she skidded under my bed to hide. Striding in seconds later, Mum thundered, "Where is she?" and I mutely surrendered, pointing at the bed. She was hauled out and spanked as I watched.

Nothing could have been more natural than for me to deny all knowledge and spare Martha ten seconds of loyalty, yet I failed—on that occasion and many others—to defend her. In my desire to fit in, not only did I surrender my preferences, but I also rarely took social risks, such as shielding my siblings from parental wrath. Slowly learning to deal with the unfairness of my physical limitations, I rarely considered the difficulties that Martha, Elouise, or Simon faced. Met with my apparent indifference, Elouise went off and did her own thing, Simon became increasingly self-reliant, and Martha very gradually grew wary and distanced herself.

Slowly, I made sense of myths surrounding me. I came to dread the presence of guests at our table. The repetition of punchy one-liners such as, "Fran was delivered by Kristof, you see, the cord was around her neck," or, "An unfortunate case of negligence, but what could we do . . . ?" accompanied the asparagus starter and the delicious beefsteak. Like all children whose parents will insist on embarrassing them in public, I squirmed in my seat and blushed. While part of me was naturally curious, I dreaded hearing what had happened to me and hated knowing that the circumstances of my birth were so often part of the table talk. Embarrassment at my physical shortcomings— as well as a fear that my brain might also be slightly broken—may have fuelled the constant reminders of my deliverance. In the ironing away of small wrinkles, I was only expected to smile. How does a young child look happy (grateful), sad (piteous), and relieved (lucky) all at once?

My mother might occasionally add, "I took you with me, you know, although they tried to persuade me that I should leave you at the hospital, put you in a home," and then resume her task of pouring, eating, wiping her lips, leaving statements such as these hovering between us like unexploded bombs. Children take what is said to them very literally. Painful half-truths thrown out over their heads without any of the love or patience that is needed to disarm them, fester with hidden threats. What was a spindle shank like me to make of this latest revelation? I felt like weeping with terror at the prospect of being abandoned, so nakedly laid out for public viewing. A precocious child might have dared to ask, "You mean . . . I should be grateful you did not abandon me?" I could not pluck up enough courage, in case her answer came back, "Yes, of course you should be grateful," which I would take to mean, "*You should be grateful because you are really such a nuisance.*" So I smiled inanely, nodded, and mumbled a useless "thank you" before resolving to be good forever and ever.

Now it comes to me with blinding clarity: I know just how lucky I am. My mother took it upon herself to rescue me, as best she could, from the million and one careless expectations of failure that would have condemned me to a life in a hospital, hidden away, a source of shame and "something we don't talk about." I now understand that my fate hung precariously for a time, held only by the single thread of Mum's determination. I came within a hair's breadth of having no life at all.

Chapter Ten

One bright, fresh morning, I was seated at the kitchen step, grimacing against the glare of the sun on my face. "Eyes open, mouth shut!" called Mum, repeating a household mantra, this one invested with the hope that eventually I would "look more normal." She was busy with her usual household tasks, unloading the car after another trip to the market. Obediently, thankful of her reminder to not look odd, I clamped shut my mouth and opened my eyes, though in the sharp morning light it hurt to do so.

"Anyway, come on!" she called, "We're going to the hospital. Have you been to the bathroom?" I slipped off my seat and pulled myself along to the car. What now? Elouise, Simon, and Martha were quite happy to be left in the care of the household staff as we drove away.

I was pleasantly surprised. Waiting for me at my hospital appointment were two gleaming elbow crutches. At five and a half years old, after crawling everywhere and pulling myself up by the arms, I was finally introduced to the world of those who walk upright, tall and thinly. I was flooded with tremors of laughter and excitement. A conqueror now, I was going places, I could do things! I would leave behind my passivity.

"Frances! Come on, Fran, you're always last, aren't you?"

"Well, *excuse me!*" I would put on my famous, non-committal smile, the one that suggested I had been listening and otherwise gave nothing away. I was sometimes not a very nice girl, but too many other concerns jumped up and moved self-importantly to the front of the queue, so that the matter with my manners was often overlooked. While everyone was told, "We don't make exceptions for Fran, we treat her just the same as everyone else," much of the time I was just trying to keep up. Martha was aware what this effort cost me, and in later years, as we walked home from school together, she would go slowly and wait patiently, encouraging, "Come on, Fran, not much further now" as I staggered and sweated.

One of the first things I did with my newfound freedom was learn to swim, first creeping and then leaping into outdoor pools where I splashed with joyful abandon. Once I learned to float, there was no need to worry that I would drown, so the cool, salty spindrift of the ocean that lifted me became my friend. Delight infused me, and it didn't matter that I swam using only my arms, which were very strong. I discovered an affinity with Popeye and his muscley biceps and I greedily ate up my spinach.

Once, I almost died by the ocean and in the process lost my carefree attitude towards open water. I was a young teenager vacationing at another beach on the Atlantic coast of Africa, where the currents are stronger and broader than I was used to. That morning, the vast tide felt surreal, as a wide expanse of flat sand stretched out to a faraway line of faintly shimmering waves. The blue seemed so distant, a mere painted smudge a hundred miles out. Very abruptly where there had been sand flats, now there was a crashing frenzy. These waves were not fresh and friendly, but hard, towering walls of water, a full-scale assault. My mother was not there to warn me and I was badly out of my depth. I stood bravely, for three seconds sizing up my chances. I knew that I had no time to outrun the pursuit, that the sheer weight of water bearing down on me was vast, thick, and as hard as rock. Offering a prayer, I took a deep breath and held on as I was engulfed in a carrying, rolling frenzy of churning waves which, thankfully, bore me up the rough sands to the shore. Trying to resist the back pull, I gripped as gravel slipped through my fingers and salty water sucked, sand buzzing in my ears and churning water tugging at my long hair. After what felt like my whole life, I surfaced to air. Snatching another breath, I mercifully reached shallow ground where I could scramble up the beach on all fours and, in a jerky panic, pull myself to safety.

The rest of the family was starting to think about lunch.

"Are you all right, Fran?" asked Elouise, coming over and draping a towel over me.

"Yes, I'm fine," I said.

Chapter Eleven

"Where are the car keys?" Father asked, his voice sharper than usual. We four children abruptly stopped our squabbles, while Mum patted her pockets. Martha was playing beside me, and Simon was building something complicated with his beloved "Meccano" set, seated near the large low window that overlooked the garden. Like cats, we scattered to the edge of the room, searching with wide eyes.

"Where are the keys?" was repeated more loudly. We tried to look busy, concerned, helpful; glancing under chairs, feeling with little hands beneath the old sofa where we discovered forgotten pencils, twisted pieces of paper, plastic "Spyrograph" disks. We wanted to be anywhere else, not in this room with that shouting.

Poor Mummy, her obvious concern seemed only to inflame Father's irritation. He may only have been thinking, "How can she be afraid of me? I've only lost the keys, and I am in such a hurry!" but some of his frustration showed in towering impatience. Though I was sitting on the sidelines, I felt a whipping resonance begin to build and sought refuge in familiar toys. Simon was darting around the room, searching under cushions, by tables, behind doors, and the long drapes. While I froze, he moved, or stood straight in front of a growing impatience directed at no one in particular. Mummy looked everywhere she could think of. No keys.

Father's working day started early, with schools and offices open from seven until one o'clock, when everything closed for lunch, and often for the rest of the day. But his day was stalling before it had started. He was stranded at home because someone had lost the keys for the car, the garage, the gate.

His fingers drummed the roof of the car. He was going to find Mummy when he felt a lump in a pocket of his trousers. Many times his hands had searched and found nothing, but suddenly: a miracle. "Estelle, I have found them!" he called, immediately happy again. She ran out to see, both relieved and dismayed when she glimpsed what he held aloft in his fingers. She could not help saying, "You could have looked there first."

"But I did. I swear I did!" Though he recovered quickly, Kristof's anger still reverberated. "I'm sorry, love, really I am! Look, I must go now, I'm late." There was a plea in his eyes as he fired up the car. "See you at lunchtime, though I may be a little late," he called.

Estelle ran back into the house where we were all in tears. She mopped our faces, murmuring consolations and wondering . . . If only she could think of a way to—"Shall we go to the beach, children?" Her gambit worked. While Elouise and Simon ran away by themselves, Martha took my arm and we walked behind them, taking our time to cross the road and go down the sand.

As Martha grew taller, more adventurous, and beautiful, I loved and admired her. At the same time, I was so jealous of her limbs' freedom. The affection that she aroused in Father was obvious and I was furious, sensitive to every tiny slight. My confused emotions did not come clean, but twisted together in a knot which lodged somewhere in my body.

How long might it take to apologize for the cruelty I inflicted on others—and on myself—because I was so unexpressed—so frustrated? Life was proving a difficult balancing act for us all, my mother and siblings particularly feeling the brunt of my frustration: damned if they tried to help me ("I can manage!"); damned if they didn't ("How could you leave me here, lagging behind you?"). I brushed their hands aside so I fell behind. They went ahead and I yearned for company. It is this contradiction—not my physical compromising—which lies at the core of my immobility.

As I felt myself pushed into aloneness, it was as if a pane of glass came down and fitted itself neatly around me. If my anger and anguish had not so often been greeted with disapproval, if I could have found more creative outlets, perhaps Martha might have escaped many small horrors from me. Perhaps more relaxed love would have soothed us all, but my parents were already too busy with so many different concerns and there were few others to notice what went on, or to care that we children should be gentler with each other.

Chapter Twelve

Christmas for the young is a magical time of glittering treasures, of indelibly bright impressions fixed forever in the putty of small minds: the rare sight of colored lights on the Christmas tree, antics during late nights, the scents of baking and spicy sweets, tangerines and ginger biscuits; a time of blessings, new beginnings, and firm resolutions for improvement. For us all, surprises waited beneath the pine tree. I have no notion how a conifer was found for us each year in Africa, but its sweet scent wafted through the living room, dark, prickly branches concealing parcels brightly wrapped and hidden for us to find early on Christmas morning.

I watched as Mummy sat at her Singer sewing machine, her open sewing box spilling pins, threads, measuring tape, and scissors. At times like these, she seemed to swim in a lake of luxurious cloth, which she fashioned into matching dresses for Martha and me. Leftover scraps were meshed into miracle pinafores of jointed stars or sewn to make dolls' nightdresses and two-piece suits complete with contrasting trim, hooks, and eyes.

Martha and I might have been almost six. That year, I felt that we were especially lucky. We were wearing new dresses made in bright patchwork. Martha was chattering happily. Filled with excitement, she and I sat playing with our dolls near the tree. Mummy had found each of us such wonderful toys.

Unknown to Martha and me, Father had accepted an invitation to tour the local children's hospital. The superintendent there was very proud of the facilities on offer and delighted that our father had agreed to honor him with a special visit on that day. Of course, Martha and I did not pick up this conversation, or collect any of its meaning, absorbed as we were in unwrapping presents.

"Here. Children, come here!" Father was anxious about something. We didn't know what. Words died on our lips and we sat anxiously rooted to the spot. Martha and I stayed very still where we had been playing. I wanted to crawl under the tree to hide. Father burst into the living room.

"Do you know where I've been, children?" he asked.

I almost said, "Yes, you have been to the bathroom," because that's where I was often told to go.

Elouise answered for us, "Yes, Father, have you visited the hospital?"

"I have just come from the hospital. You know what I saw there?" He was loud, like a horse at a gallop. "I saw children who have no toys. They have nothing, they do not even have shoes to wear, or blankets for the beds, or combs or . . . or anything. It's Christmas, they have nothing!" Father's grief was making him incoherent. Mum went over and whispered comfort, but in his anguish he brushed her off.

Like an actor in a play, Father swept forward, bearing down on Martha and me who, failing totally to understand that any of this sorrow might have anything to do with us, had the impudence to look so happy together.

"You have so much!" he was shouting. "You have so many toys, we must give some of them to the children at the hospital, and I will take them, straight away!"

We greeted his suggestion with shock and disbelief. On this day of all days, to make us part with toys we had only just received? Impossible! Before he could be calmed, father was pulling toys out of cupboards, away from under the tree, and out of small hands. We were all thinking, this cannot really be happening, because our mummy has just given us these toys.

"So, you do not want to give up your presents? Then—then you must give up—*these!*" Carried away by the part he was playing, he targeted our favorite dolls nestled in our arms. "One of you must give up your doll! Fran? Is it to be you? No? Then, Martha—you!" And her own precious friend was pulled and swept out of her reach, into a pile on the floor, like an offering on a tearful bonfire.

Martha cried out, "No! Please, not Millie! She's my favorite!" Indeed, her doll was very pretty, with blond wool plaits, cornflower blue eyes in a soft stitched face, and a blue smock with careful petticoats. She was far more beautiful than either of my rag dolls, who were ragged indeed. But there was no reprieve for Martha, or for Millie. I sat rigid, clutching my Mopsy. We were all crying noisily by now, a sound guaranteed to send my father's anxiety into orbit. Mummy sat in frozen disbelief, her face rigid and paling with shock.

I was allowed to keep my doll and I felt guilty for many months at this glaring favoritism, which filled me with a sick feeling. Martha was inconsolable over her loss even though I offered her one of my dolls. Of course, hers was the most beautiful by far of the clutch that we held between us and set down to tea parties. I knew this and felt Martha's injustice. I could have helped her by giving up my doll at Christmas. Deep inside, I knew I would have coped better. Where possessions are concerned, I am usually more robust and would have recovered more quickly, whereas it took many months for the pain of Martha's loss to recede. It would not be the last time that Martha would shield me from suffering. Much worse was in store for her in years to come.

The following Christmas, my mother purchased for Martha a very grand plastic doll which walked when held by the hand, cried when filled with water, and, for all I knew, did cartwheels when no one was looking. From the moment I clapped eyes on it, I was filled with insane jealousy: this doll could do things that I couldn't, and in my childish egoism, I believed the family was mocking me. Dear Mum was only trying to console my sister with the best doll she could find.

My father could not help noticing the distressing contrast our affluence offered to the lives of others. Unfortunately, I watched and drew the wrong conclusions, vowing that if such unhappiness was what money brought, I would never want to be rich. In my own way, I took an oath of poverty. Only recently did I see how successfully I have carried this resolution with me through my life.

Chapter Thirteen

As part of the business of diplomacy, our parents were invited to many formal functions. Some invitations, which always took priority over our usual family arrangements, inevitably dropped into the social calendar at short notice and Mum quickly became an expert at dressing up in five minutes to go out for the evening. Even so, Father made sure that whenever we could, we all ate meals together, especially after we children had mastered the use of knives and forks, could feed ourselves fried eggs without smearing our faces and when I was able to sit up straight in my seat.

Our mealtimes were punctuated by lively conversations. Obscure theories around any subject seemed to catch my parents' attention: politics, religion, languages, or physics, anything was open for debate.

Many eyes watched us daily as, around a dining table covered with spotless linen and laid with gilt china dishes, delicious meals were served. The drama of yet another discussion unfolded with the napkins, at first quietly and with attention to detail, then gradually with more stains, smears, and crumpling. Mutual understanding and politeness seemed to evaporate as our food grew cold, sharpness and annoyance taking the place of gentle discourse. Perhaps this is one reason I prefer plain food: rich fare feels argumentative to me, as if spicy meatballs in tomato sauce may start an attack of indigestion.

Our parents' impatience seemed to unfurl slowly, at first so politely, that to begin with I did not feel any of the sharpness that ricocheted between them. I watched smilingly, unable to understand the words flying overhead. Politely, we were reminded of the importance of table manners—"Pass the salt please, Elouise; sit up straight, Fran." For what it was worth, I learned that when we were with Mummy, our hands were to be hidden in our laps. When with Father, our wrists should rest on the table, which seems more polite, otherwise what might hands be doing under the table?

There were servants serving, listening, taking instructions, asking questions, and seeking advice. Despite our daily audience, anyone gathering a peck of courage to join in the banter had best beware. Regularly, one of us would leave the table in a flurry of tears. Luckily, because Martha and I were the youngest, our contributions were mostly discounted. The heavy guns were reserved for Mum, Elouise, and Simon.

Father was at his most entertaining during breakfast, amusing and kind; he was often in charge, while Mummy roused herself more gently. Martha and I stifled our joy at his endless joking, which he knew we adored. To the accompaniment of our prattling, "Lake Titicaca" became one of our favorite wheezes, our key to a private land of gasping, aching laughter.

Left to my own devices, I was as guilty as anyone of the usual pranks and mischief. "Come on!" I cried to the others one morning after breakfast, "I know a really good game."

They looked curiously in my direction.

"Let's run around the table, and each time we go around, we have to grab a handful of cornflakes and stuff them in our mouths. We have to finish each handful before we get to the next."

"Okay!" A chime of consent as the gallop began, as they ran and I staggered gamely round and round the long table. We snatched at dry cereal, cramming crispy curls messily into our mouths. Because they were dry, the cornflakes tasted toasty delicious, though they were difficult to swallow, which was a big part of the challenge. We were enjoying paroxysms of delight, when Mum marched into the room.

"What are you doing!" she shouted, incredulously.

"Well, you see, Mummy, you have to run around the table . . ." I was so wound up with happiness that I was shaking all over and could hardly get my words out, but the thread of my story died as I looked up, and saw her frown and survey the mess we had made: the litter of squashed food, dirtied tableware, sodden flakes all over the floor, and the empty cereal box which told its own guilty story.

"That was a brand new box!" she cried, "You have wasted a whole box." I was sorry for the damage, for the fact that this latest expensive import had such an ignominious end, yet nothing could dismantle my joy at sharing such gleeful abandon with Simon, Martha, and Elouise. It was so rare that we were all happy together. That joy lived on with me for years, battling my sense of shame at my naughtiness. Glee won in the end. The game was worth it.

Not everything was funny. One morning I watched through a door left ajar my mother weeping in abject grief. She was sitting in the master bedroom on a low stool, hunched forward and clutching at her dress, as if to pull it over her knees and down her legs for protection. Father was shouting. Suddenly it seemed that tense discomfort could be felt in lots of places—at mealtimes, on the terrace. I knew that Mum's grief was undeserved, but I was unsure what I could do.

Chapter Fourteen

Father's current tour of duty in Africa was ending. Meanwhile, we heard whisperings about a man called Idi Amin who was living dangerously close by and who had expelled all the Asians from Uganda. Mother decided that now would be a good time for her and Father to separate. She would not be following her husband to his next posting, so he would have to take up the responsibilities of foreign work and travel alone.

My parents faced a dilemma familiar to all diplomatic families: whether to bring the whole family along on the career path of the main wage earner, tackling the difficulties of travelling, constant upheaval, and unpredictable schooling along the way, or whether to opt for a more settled existence. My father's travels took him across the world, to Canada, to Europe, to Angola, and Rwanda, to Costa Rica, and Croatia. Perhaps aware of my particular dependence on her, my mother chose to move back to Scotland permanently. She decided that all her children must come home with her, so that we could go to school, settle down, and study. After that move in December 1972, we no longer lived all together as a family unit, except on rare occasions during the holidays.

There was also some talk of taking me home to get me looked at; I was going to have operations to make me better. Of course, I didn't really understand what that meant, only that the shape of my feet was going to change. So I hugged my legs and feet, talked to them, and swore that I loved them. I sat cross-legged on the floor hoping that I could stay put.

While Mum was laying plans, we were playing at the beach and swimming in the ocean. I sat and watched the wide sky. We went on a safari where I looked up at giraffes as they licked and munched high-up leaves carefully, dipping their heads from great heights. We took excursions to the hills where the climate is so cool that the grass only grows in short blades, like those of a well-tended English lawn. Perhaps these treats were my father's way of saying goodbye to us and of expressing hope in his choices. Rarely, in those last, drifting days did Mummy and Father do things together, although shared meal times remained a fixture. With us, our parents were kind, distracted by more pressing difficulties.

Our bush baby, a tiny primate pet with huge eyes and hair like a dandelion clock that stood up on his back, had lived in a semi-wild state with us and was left to fend for itself among the colonies of its kin that had their home in the trees in the grounds of the house. Our gentle dogs were re-homed and they howled at parting with us. I broke my promise not to leave them. Martha and I also had to leave behind our enormous yellow teddies, so we all howled together in one noisy mess.

I am grateful for my life abroad, even one marred with arguments, anger, and a cloying sense of being cosseted because I was a privileged, white, disabled girl. I am grateful that I have been able to live with wildness all around me, to feel the freedom of great spaces. I feel blessed for having seen large elephants sauntering across unfenced roads. For the leaping impala and the watchful crested crane, I give thanks. In the music, laughter, movement, and color, in the brightness of the big country, I discovered how wonderful life can be. Africa's vibrant reality helped me to remember that there is a reason to hold faith with heaven. Knowing this is what saved me in the gray years.

Chapter Fifteen

The airplane touched down in the afternoon darkness of mid-winter. Dozy children with dollies and rucksacks clambered down high steps, in the face of a cool drizzle, muffled against the wind. We felt chilled and sleepy. Where were we? Trudging along corridors, our thin canvas shoes slipped on smooth concrete and along white corridors; unfamiliar lines of glass, metal, and smooth plastic. After travelling thousands of miles, our tans already looked bleached out under the strip lights of the airport.

We were bundled into a taxi and driven through the narrow, dim streets of Edinburgh to stay with Grandma and Grandpa.

"Come in, dears, I have the fire on!" greeted Eleanor at her narrow porch. "Leave your things here just now. Come in."

Against the rain, the front door slammed heavily as Martha and I looked at each other in bewilderment. We gazed around the small hallway; saw the wall-to-wall carpeting, the close banisters, and thick wooden doors. Everything looked and smelled different: roses and wood polish. In the corner of the living room to our left, we glimpsed a television set, green and red, showing a football match. This we had not seen before and we gawked, peering through the crack of the open door.

Above me, Grandma was speaking, her tones remembered, yet unfamiliar. "We will be having something to eat soon, and then I am afraid that it will be time for the twins to go to bed. Martha? Frances?

Come and meet Grandpa." She ushered us in, over strange softness that muffled our footsteps.

Eleanor and Stuart had visited us several times while we were living abroad. Grandma's deep, gentle voice was what I remembered first, before I looked up again into her blue eyes and admired the sheen of her white wavy hair. She smiled widely and hugged each of us in turn, her daughter last.

As I grew older, it became clearer to me that Eleanor was gentle but often frustrated. She spoke quietly, yet beneath her composed and compromising exterior, she hid real fire. It had been her hope that if her daughters studied hard, they could make something of themselves; take the opportunities she missed and escape to the soaring hills that seemed to beckon. Eleanor spent too much time at the kitchen sink with her back to the chat, resigned or unhappy, working with her hands.

In my mind's eye, I see Grandma cooking to "make ends meet," rarely with glee. In Eleanor, there lived a smooth, fragrant beauty, and I longed to be caught in her arms and swung round. Sadly, she had little time for such playfulness and instead tied in her enthusiasms with her apron strings, pulling herself down with grim determination to the tasks she was left with: she might fetch a small block of cheese, a single very large potato, and, using a cauliflower bought cheaply from the local greengrocer because it was on the turn, produce the most amazing meal, with the minimum of fuss. Her husband's sullen terror of enduring another poverty like in 1931, meant they rarely ate in a restaurant or traveled abroad and that Stuart kept by him the same pair of spectacles for over thirty years, answering shortly to my mother's incredulity: "They are just fine!"

Occasionally, Eleanor could be discovered clutching a piece of dark chocolate, which she consumed secretively while apologizing for her extravagance. And every so often in their later years, when it became apparent that neither Grandma nor Grandpa would actually starve, she purchased a pair of season tickets and took one of her grown granddaughters out to the local concert hall for the evening. At such times, when choosing to exercise her elegant personal preferences, Eleanor shone and glimmered like a queen. She wore beautiful clothes when she had occasion to. She spoke kindly to everyone she met. When she wasn't at home, she felt free and stretched her wings wide.

And so here on the doorstep, there came her elder daughter back to her, bringing four straggling children filled with tales of travel, all misty-eyed and asking strange questions. Would this be counted a victory or a defeat?

We were "back home" in the city where Mum grew up, arriving the week before Christmas, two weeks before our eighth birthday. Wet, cold, and windy weather beat over my face and legs. I tried to like it; I tried to enjoy my first Christmas and New Year in the dark climate for which Christmas lights are intended. The first time I encountered slippery December rain beating at the slant I piped up, "Grandma, is this the rainy season?" to which she laughingly answered, "Oh no, dear! It rains here all the time."

Chapter Sixteen

Overnight, Mum's priorities changed. From organizing formal receptions and parties to overseeing catering and deliveries in unpredictable timetables, she effectively began the life of a single parent, with four children to provide and cater for on a minimal budget. Despite arrangements with my father that would not have left her penniless, the costs of our care forever emptied her bank account: new shoes, clothes, and an ever-mounting food bill must have left her wondering what she could do next. For the first time, she had to earn money. Setting set up her new home, it was agreed that she would take over and eventually purchase Grandma and Grandpa's house, while they moved to a bungalow further out of the city, with a wonderful back garden where Grandma spent all her spare moments.

Elouise had already started boarding at a large coeducational school in the Scottish countryside. It was straightforward for Simon to also pass the entrance examination and begin there the following year, which meant that only Martha and I remained at home. The house had space for Mum to start a business from the front room, and she ran a series of successful ventures that gave her enough of an income to live comfortably, providing she was careful. Meantime, she had Martha and me to look after.

Grandma gave me extra lessons to make sure I could add, spell, and write, though of course I was taught all these subjects at school. I don't recall my siblings having to sit patiently indoors while the sun shone, counting or writing. Perhaps they saw me sitting idle and considered I could be doing something useful. My elders may have concluded that, at the very least, I should be given extra help as an insurance policy against any grain of latent stupidity that might be lurking in my head. Okay, so I couldn't figure out math, which was like a foreign language to me, but so what? I wasted hours and years of my time at school and later at university, deliberately studying difficult subjects and trying to understand the incomprehensible, precisely because I felt under pressure to prove I was not stupid, by which I mean "mentally retarded," the phrase in universal use at the time.

When my mother was considering which schools might be suitable for us, she was caught unaware by this prejudice.

"I'm dreadfully sorry, Mrs. Freyerling, but we cannot *possibly* give your daughter a place at our school. We have the reputation of our girls to consider. We *cannot* lower the tone!" declared one headmistress with delusions of grandeur. I wonder how Martha must have felt when she learned that she was refused entry because her sister was disabled. Such stories as these Mum shared with me, pointed out attitudes of which I had been blissfully ignorant, and fuelled a growing desire to oblige others.

To begin with, we were enrolled in the nearby school, the same one my daughter now attends. Seline is much happier there than I was. Martha and I were left to become acclimatized by ourselves and I was completely disorientated. I could barely understand the system of all-day schooling, though I gradually made more sense of the new timetables designed for a day that began at nine, rather than seven in the morning, and finished at three, rather than at lunchtime. Everything felt strange and looked different. I was not used to seeing bars on the walls of the playground and the separate entrances for boys and girls. Our hard-to-place accents marked Martha and me out, though no one wanted to know how different it had been for us before, so despite all the children milling around, I rarely spoke or played.

When Mummy saw how lost I was in the new system, she hit on the wonderful idea of enrolling us at the local Steiner school. With its relaxed attitude to learning, creative curriculum, and wonderful gardens, it was easier for me, at any rate, to settle into. Foreign languages, songs, poetry, and art were a big part of our lessons, and the teachers seemed less concerned about me singing in class . . . Two of our neighbors were at the same school, so we had new friends to play with. Gradually, I came out of my shell.

In the cold wind and rain, I ached and hobbled. Despite the chill we were always playing outside, and over time, Martha and I grew more used to the changeable climate. I came to love the sounds of our new home: the whistle of a lone blackbird at dusk, the heavy sighing of large broadleaf trees in the wind. The moving seasons, with their bursts of sharp, poignant coloring, helped me to notice that bad things pass and change brings hope and renewal. Even as I hunched my shoulders beneath slate-gray, glowering skies on cold days, my eyes began to distinguish muted madders, russet, gold glimmers of gorse, and lavender hues of heather in the hills.

After the shock of winter and the delay of an eagerly awaited spring, the long, sunny days and light nights of summer felt wonderful. In the years before cars took up all the space and made side roads dangerous, the streets around our house became our playground. Martha and I spent long, lazy weeks laughing and playing outside, going indoors only to eat and sleep. The neighborhood children became our friends and with them I was very happy. I could do lots of things: I clambered easily and arm wrestled boys three times my size. We were harking back to earlier freedoms as we chanted songs with a skipping rope—I took up my place as chief rope turner. We threw marbles along the gutters, chalked up hopscotch, spun hoops around our waists, and played catch and tag games like "British Bulldogs." We chatted on doorsteps, ate illicit popsicles, and cadged sweets from children with liberal parents who didn't care so much about tooth decay and diabetes.

My mother seemed to hold her own views, often reminding me how embarrassing I was being, or how I should draw as little attention to myself as I could. As I grew older, my physical differences became harder for me to ignore. Children who didn't know me giggled, whispered, stared, and pointed. They yelled obscenities in my direction while their mothers pulled in their skirts and strode past, leaving me lots of room. They told their children "Don't stare!" and avoided my eyes. They didn't see my polite smile and they probably didn't realize that I understood everything they said.

Chapter Seventeen

There was no great fanfare, no party when I left my elbow crutches behind and walked independently. I simply outgrew them and they were not replaced. Perhaps I should not say "walk" since I shuffled along, often launching my body by sheer bravado. Once I learned to run, I fell often and knocked my head repeatedly, but I didn't let that stop me. Like a coiled spring, I had lots of energy and was always on the move. I liked to play the horse and, with a rope thrown around my midriff, I could pull Martha along the road on her roller skates, though sometimes I could hardly stand while laughing. We went fast as I was a good runner, light and flying. It was easy, of course, and there was a trick: after the first tug, the skates glided smoothly.

Thankfully I never saw myself running or walking, even in the glass of shop windows. I was too busy concentrating, and in any case, my gait was too jolting to allow for much introspection. The single drawback of increased mobility was that, to keep my balance, I moved fast. I became clumsier and more accident prone. Bumping into chairs, I knocked over lamps and pulled cloths off tables as I rushed through a room. Anything left lying in my path tripped me up. China and glass were often dropped and there were a great many finger marks decorating the walls of our house.

Crashing down was routine, and my mother got used to telephone calls telling her I had been in an accident. It became something of a joke between us. While everyone else would be in a panic, Mum and I became quite resigned to my injuries, bruises, and stitches, and we would usually be able to laugh about them. What happened at Rosemary's party was a rather spectacular example.

If you could have seen me that afternoon at school, you would have noticed my wide grin. For once, just like everyone else, I had received an invitation to Rosemary's birthday party! I loved Rosemary, a kind girl with dark hair who wore pretty dresses and smiled a lot. Her party was fabulous, like a fantasy dream, with bright balloons of painted faces, fizzy jelly, and ice cream. Happiness bubbles popped in clapping hands all around me.

I was rushing, when suddenly a vast oil-fired radiator was lying on top of me. It had crashed down on my head, although I didn't hear a thing. My foot just pulled a cord and it toppled. Oops! Scorching metal scored lines over my face and pale burns on my hands.

As I was carried away and laid with great tenderness on the sofa in the front room, someone read me snippets from *Charlie and the Chocolate Factory* while the party evaporated. Telephone calls were made to locate my mother and, when the phone rang without reply, questions were asked: where was she? I said to try my grandparents' house and gave the number. My hosts were impressed. Later at the hospital, while I was being patched up, the young gentle doctor saw that the impact had dented my skull and torn a gash over my eye socket. Aware that my beauty was at stake and that the anesthetic he had pumped in to my forehead with his very long needle gave him plenty of time, he worked with patient hands and intense concentration, very carefully sewing in twelve stitches.

The next Monday at school, I scuffed unsteadily over playground concrete cracked by uneven tree roots. I was given hugs and some extra presents. Susan came up and linked arms with me. My head was throbbing, numb and wrapped in a very large bandage that came over my forehead to protect the delicate stitching around my eye. There were rainbow bruises on the rest of my face and burn scalds over my hands.

As I left the school gates that day with a special balloon that Rosemary herself had given me and tied gently around my hand, Nicky—charming and slippery and taller than the rest of us—sidled along the railings and popped my balloon. For good measure, just to make sure that I knew how much he hated all the attention I was getting, he unleashed a long gout of spit, which he had obviously been working in his mouth. It landed on that little part of my cheek that was not bandaged. I stood unsteadily, sweating with distress, crying small tears.

Chapter Eighteen

Shortly after our return to Britain, Mum began to consult medical opinion in earnest about my condition and the prospects for its improvement. As a young girl in whom others appeared interested, at first I was very happy to show how well I could walk, and enthusiastically strutted my stuff, as pleased as Punch to show off, "See what I can do!" In pale, antiseptic rooms peopled by stiff professionals sporting starched whites and wearing detached frowns of concentration, I obliged repeated requests to take off shoes and socks and pull myself across shiny hospital floors.

Where I came from and according to the manners I had been taught at home, a frown was a prelude to a telling off: there must have been something wrong. I wondered what it could be. No one seemed to talk to me directly, they just looked, with blank-faced concentration, and consulted in mumbles with each other or with my mother. They spoke at me as if issuing instructions to a machine. What were they thinking? I hardly knew.

As months and years accumulated and I was *still* being asked to show myself off, this slipping stagger of mine became a loathsome burden that I was forced to share and display with total strangers, whether I liked it or not. I became a hostile, angry teenager and when that made no difference, I retreated so far into depression that the smiling, happy girl I had been at seven completely disappeared.

She and I had a long way to go. After the socks and shoes and the walking demonstration, I was often asked to quickly remove all my outer clothing and haul myself up onto a slippery couch for a lengthy consultation. Lots of lying back for bends, stretches, pulls, and pushes, mumbled instructions, which I worked to obey: "Can you raise your leg, reach my hand if I put it up here?" or "Now, try to push against my hand as hard as you can." I tried as hard as I could and made it into a challenge or a game, just for a bit of interest. "And again?" Yes, okay. Notes were made on a pad, or whispered into a machine. There may still be a stack of papers ten feet high stored in hospital archives from here to London, for all I know.

After being given a lengthy once over, trying not to feel embarrassed by cold hands, coat flaps in the way, at my dirty or torn undergarments exposed to view, I was allowed to get dressed, while discussion— always over my head—continued. I was not allowed time off for good behavior and my discharge papers never arrived. There was nothing I could say. I had no words, yet, for what I was feeling and I didn't know if it would be polite to disagree or ask them to explain to me what was being suggested. So I lay back on the couch and it went on.

If I'd had a say in it, I would have liked to not sit in half-clothed vulnerability on a couch, my legs dangling beneath me. A tall, self-possessed woman, my friend and mentor, would be in the room with me and her presence at my side would garner me some new respect. She would raise me up and ensure I had space to dress in peace and join her at my leisure. She would give me as much time as I needed, to speak slowly so that all the doctors would understand. I'd be given a comfortable chair to sit on and lots of room to think and breathe, and this is what I would say:

"My legs and feet are beloved to me. We have grown together in companionable peace. We have found a success, which admittedly may not be your usual stepping ease. I find walking comfortable enough and usually pain-free. So why are you talking about me?"

They may have answered, "We are having a chat, dear. It's nothing for you to worry about."

And I would have liked to challenge them: "I know. But what are you saying? That I need to be fixed?"

"We are trying to make you better."

"Better than what? Better than I am now? You do not like my walking? Can you explain?"

"Well, you might find that difficult to understand. Trust us."

"Try me."

"Well, we were just explaining to your mother that, in layman's terms (what is a layman?) we are going to cut you open, rearrange the lie of your bones, and stitch you back together again. If that doesn't work, we can try something else."

"I see."

"And then you will walk more easily, you see?"

"You think."

"Yes, we are fairly certain we can help you to walk better."

"But you don't know for sure."

"No—well, no one does, really."

After a pause, during which I would feel the warmth of support at my side from my tall friend, I would answer, "I think I understand you, but let me see if I've got this straight. You are trying to make me better and so you will cut at me and slash at my feet and sew and hope. Have I got that right?"

"Well, there's a bit more to it than that, actually."

"But you are proposing to pull at my roots and cut my feet, in the hope that the 'new me' you plant in the ground can make a better go of it, than I have managed so far?"

"Essentially, yes."

Then I would quietly explain to all the gathered company of men in white coats, that whether they could see this or not, *there is nothing wrong with me. I don't feel different from you, or in need of mending. God made me as I am. I can walk. I feel well. I do not require any more well-meaning meddling on my behalf.*

When they had heard what I wanted to say, I'd shake my head in disbelief that they would consider that such a thing as *what I look like when I walk* mattered. Then I would get up, shake hands goodbye, and leave behind their horrible smelly rooms forever. My tall friend, my mum, and I are going outside for a walk in the park and then home to eat ice cream and watch television together—so there!

But no tall woman was sitting beside me. There was my small mother, looking by turns angry and unsure.

Chapter Nineteen

As I inched taller, grew less sweet, and progressed to gangly and embarrassing, "Project Frances" took on a new twist: I was to go into hospital. That is where all these discussions were leading. For me, this was a new adventure.

When I was nine, one day, in accordance with hospital regulations, a small suitcase was packed with all I needed for a three-week stay: my nightie, dressing gown, slippers—which I refused to wear— toothbrush, toothpaste, a bar of soap, hairbrush, teddy bear, and a change of clothes. Mum drove me to the local orthopedic hospital, which was "world famous." "Yes" she explained, "named after a princess!" She winked as she called, "Here we are! Out you get."

It was only as the car tires scrunched in the gravel car park that I realized this was not going to be fun. The vast hospital complex loomed: shabby, dirty white with tall chimneys in need of a coat of paint. Mum took my suitcase from the trunk in one hand and tucked my wrist protectively under her other arm. Ducking out of the summer sunshine into the gloom, we began the walk along corridors; long, high, endless gray corridors smelling of urine, cooked cabbage, toilet bleach, and antiseptic. We walked quickly, while I admired the shine on the floor and resisted the urge to run headlong—I liked running. Slightly breathless with fear, I was thinking, "What joy . . . if I could just sit down here, hook up my legs over one arm, and spin around on my bottom like I used to, on the warm wooden floors of our old house." Waltzing gleefully round and round, that was the nearest I have ever come to real dancing.

Mum and I turned into Ward One, the children's ward at the far end of a very long corridor. The room was large, bright, and airy, with French windows that were opened up on fine days to let fresh air and sunshine in. Boys' beds were on one side of a partition running the length of the room, girls' on the other side. That was some scheme for keeping youth safe, which could only have been dreamt up by an anemic civil servant who had no children of his own to torment. What if, unlike me, you spent months in a hospital? What then, for the happy mixing of boys and girls? My bed was at the end of the ward and on this, my first stay, there was deep unfamiliarity in being there: I knew I was not ill. Perhaps I had landed on a planet with private, unknown rituals. Strange smells brought on nausea.

My mother was leaving. As she was dropping me off, hospital visiting hours were over, though we would find out that in the children's ward, parents were not asked to leave, but allowed to come and go much as they wished. Mum would be back tomorrow. I knew she would, she was faithful. After she had gone, I felt crumbly inside, and tried not to cry. There was no anger: I understood that all this was going to make me better. Feeling shaky and unsure, I held myself in and looked around the room. I saw faces crooked up at me, eyes smiling, and headed off to investigate. I would be fine, as soon as I knew what happened next.

I unpacked my bits and pieces and a nurse showed me where to put them. I slipped off the bed, away to explore as there seemed to be no one telling me I couldn't. I jaunted away and soon discovered the large toy room near the entrance of the ward, crammed with shelves stocked with bright playthings, books, and comics I didn't get at home. That made me smile and laugh. Look! Jackie annuals, Beano, Beezer! This cupboard I got to know very well. The bright books became my friends, letting me into an amazing world of naughty children, glamour, action, excited teen sweethearts, and seventies pop idols. Color, action, love.

The next morning we were roused at six. My ordinary clothes had been thoughtfully tidied away, and at the foot of the bed I discovered a hospital gown of the sort I would wear for the rest of my stay. Shapeless garments that tied quickly at the neck and could be easily changed and washed were common sense, but becoming accustomed to wearing smelly overalls next to naked skin was another signal of my personal surrender. After a breakfast that sat queasy in my stomach, we spent ages just sitting or lying on our beds doing nothing. Hospital radio came on as soon as we woke, with its cheerful mix of requests and chart toppers.

"Why do we have to get up so early?" I asked. I was not an early bird.

"Because there's lots to do!" was their answer, though in truth we were roused early because there was lots for *everyone else* to be getting on with. We patients had to be ready to go whenever "they" wanted to see us. We waited at the beck and call of other people. We waited for a man to come and take us on a gurney or in a wheelchair to X-ray, physicals, tests, consultations, what have you. One of us might wait all day without food, because it was written on the chart at the foot of the bed, "Operation tomorrow," though there was no guarantee these would happen on schedule.

I know now that my first operation was intended to stretch my left foot with bone grafts taken from my hip; and to pin my right ankle flat to the ground. For these incursions, a surgeon drew lines over my body with a big, fat black ink pen, while I lay on a couch in a room full of people, so they could see clearly where they were going to cut me open and rearrange me. "Here, here, and here," he murmured, as the tip of the pen over my skin smelled vaporous and the tickle made me giggle. I repeated in parrot fashion, "I am going to have an operation!" as only a trusting nine-year-old can. I thought I understood what it meant.

The day before, I had no food to eat after supper at five. As part of the ritual of preparation, in the middle of the night I was woken from slumbering with some subdued chat and offered two slices of hot buttered white toast by a pretty night nurse, who walked quietly and shimmered in the shadows. Her hair was all done up so neat, she looked as if she was holding herself together with shiny pins and starched linen. The medications the next morning made me drowsy. Anesthetic tasted of floating tingles and silver tar. Count backwards from ten to one. Oblivion.

Rising up into feeling and sharp shards of sunlight hurting my eyes—pain—I feel pain with every numb twitch, beneath eyes glued shut by sleeping and a mouth as dry as the biggest desert ever. I ask for water and win a tiny sip. I can't sit up though I want to. Sharp needles in every bump and stretch. Stickiness and stuck-in-a-box plaster wafting strange hot smells. I see my mother, seated beside the bed, wearing her fur coat and clasping the rim of a sick bowl while I throw up repeatedly: too much anesthetic, a long, worrying operation. There are whispered consultations and worried glances in my direction. No tears are allowed really—mustn't embarrass people—but they will let me off this time. Faint disapproval crowds round with twinges of pin-sharp pain, angular hurts, unfamiliar.

Days passed. We hospital children were lifted and carried as the beds were stripped and clean white, crisp sheets folded and tucked in. I watched the ritual of hospital corners while, in the fresh air of the real world beyond our windows, I caught glimpses of beauty unfurling in bright sunshine.

Visitors were encouraged, as they raised the children's morale and family carers could help with feeding, tidying, and small acts of kindness. Grandma came and sat quietly by the bed, gently asking me if I was being good. On one visit she left me a box of sweets, which I could hardly believe were all for me.

Chapter Twenty

Being in the hospital had one compensation: all the patients had something "wrong" with them, so in that environment I was not so unusual. At home, rather than venturing out in public and facing the pain of being noticed for all the wrong reasons, I hid my confusion and increasingly cut myself off from other people.

I became very good at "having parties" by myself. First, I would put on the radio or music from a homemade cassette of mixed favorites. Then, I would retrieve my bundle of what passed for "knitting" or crochet. If it was a nice day, I and my radio would move to a deck chair in the back garden. I would fetch a drink, a snack, and a book or two, and that was me sorted for the next couple of hours. My mother would see what I was up to and understand, "You are having a party, aren't you?" I would nod happily and sink back blissfully in the sunshine. When, pleased with my initiative, she recounted these occasions to her mother, Eleanor would mutter, "That child has too many things," failing to understand that I was merely making the best of a difficult situation.

It is a flaw in me, perhaps, that I started listening to criticism; and my fatal mistake was to believe unkind remarks and try to learn from them. Mockery masqueraded as reason, often cloaking itself in words like "sensible," "decent," "normal," and "ordinary." The tone was reasonable. In this way, unkindness and hostility were hidden in social expectations of good behavior. So, a passing boy could insult me on the street, and because it was the street, I had to behave properly and not get cross with him or answer back.

There hovered many expectations: that I should be grateful and happy; that I should work hard; be good; not get in the way; make a point of being helpful, understanding, sympathetic to others, easy to please, and no bother. I should shun shortcuts ("Typical Frances, always trying to find the easy way to do everything!"). Had puritanism come to stay with us? Were we in agreement with those people who walked by on the other side of the road muttering, "Ah well, the sins of the fathers . . ."?

The strain of having to pretend that I was happy being constantly watched and criticized, being quietly sidelined from choices, from ordinary fooling around, and making mistakes; the wretched frustration I endured because I was getting used to the sound of only one record—"I can't"—was beginning to tell. I chewed my nails constantly down to the quick as well as my fingers and the pads of my hands, so they were a bleeding mess. I pried skin off the soles of my feet until I could hardly stand. I pulled my hair out, scratched my head until it bled, and hoped that none of this showed. Because in learning to see myself through the eyes of my critics, I had discovered it was only those things "I could not do" that I wanted to do. I was forever asking, "Why me?"

I never thought that there might be some who would look past my obvious differences to my smiling effort and be cheered by what I could achieve. I was embarrassed by myself and I tried to hide, to obliterate my difference. Of course, that was impossible. Criticism spoke loudest to me. I held my hands tightly over my ears to block out the soft song of my soul, which whispered words of beauty and hope. Instead, I spent the next decades trying ever harder to be what others wanted me to be: "normal" and for heaven's sake, not the "wee funny" that my mother seemed to fear I might become. I tried to be inconspicuous. Since that way lies madness, I wished that the ground I so frequently encountered would open up and swallow me, or better still, that I had never been born.

Chapter Twenty-One

After two years of living at home and going to the Steiner school, Mum decided to send Martha and me to a closeted learning establishment for young ladies in a nearby suburb. For the average student, our new school was roughly a twenty-five-minute walk from our house. Swinging off the bars, or jumping rope, our friends often slung across the question, "Why are you boarders?" or "Why don't you live at home?" Martha and I got used to answering, "We don't know." Often that was enough to stifle their curiosity for the time being. If my sister and I were feeling confident, we might go further and explain, "Because it's cheaper if we board. Our father's work pays the fees," an answer that was also accepted largely without comment. Our friends, not really friends, would soon move away in search of more interesting things to do.

I am glad it didn't occur to me to answer, "Because our mother does not want us at home." What could I have said if someone had then asked, "Why does your mum not want you at home?" They came very close sometimes, with, "Why don't you live with your mummy?" but I was okay with that. I could easily convince myself that none of these questions required me to answer, "Because she doesn't understand me," or "Because I don't think she loves me enough."

My mother believed she was doing us—that is, me in particular—a favor by sending us to boarding school. Perhaps she was—the jury is still out, though I know that I must take much of the blame for our predicament. At home, my sister and I had a close, often claustrophobic relationship. The sound of our arguing, mostly me in a bad mood, must have driven my mother to distraction. What a shame it was that, once again, Martha was expected to suffer alongside me.

In some ways, Martha and I were certainly better off living among other children. We had lots more opportunities to eat cakes, sweets, and jam and to do normal things like watch television, munch on chips, and read comics, few of which pleasures were allowed at home.

To their credit, the ladies who looked after us went to considerable pains to try to ensure that my sister and I slept in different dormitories so that we made our own friends. This was commendable, though often it meant that my sister was bullied on my account and I never found out. One girl, who could be quite kind to me, apparently tormented Martha daily by threatening, "Tonight, I'm going to come and beat you up!" and Martha just waited with mounting dread for lights out and the darkness that could signal an attack. She was quite unable to fight back, possibly because I had already taught her so well how to be a doormat. Maybe Martha also felt ashamed, though she needn't have. I do feel ashamed though, because it seems to me that my oddities landed us both in that quiet version of hell.

Some of the girls we were shacked up with could be very cruel, with taunting, hair pulling, and whisperings against some unlucky roommate. They knew how to be sweet when anyone in charge was watching, so they rarely got into trouble. I started out a bully too, though I soon had that pressed out of me. It wasn't only the bullying that flattened me: the school routine was relentless. The deadening, closeted regime was the very worst thing for someone already muted and stopped up with so many restrictions and neuroses.

The most difficult thing I had to endure was not the stream of snide remarks, nor even "being unusual," the exception to every girlish dream; it was not the constant ignominy of being chosen last in team games, hanging around like a spare part, forced to watch with a false smile while other people ran and jumped and played together.

It was not that I had to go to bed much earlier than my classmates, since I slept in a downstairs dormitory with younger children. It was not the chronic shortage of food or the lack of familiar contacts, apart from dear Martha. It was not the strange narrow-framed beds, the thin, lumpy candlewick covers. The worst was not at the onset of menstruation, having to wait in a queue for other girls who didn't bother to show up for their morning wash but who had "bagged" the toilet before me, so that I stood mute and desperate with my legs crossed outside the bathroom door as blood poured freely down my legs. It was not the oddness of the feelings that assailed me. It was the dancing.

The dancing? How could that be the worst thing? I don't blame you for asking, because no one at school saw much cruelty in this either, and they had many years to observe my sorrow. I was brave. I hummed the tunes. I tapped my foot. I tried not to feel in the way. Firing up a new pretense that I was perfectly happy to watch, I pasted on a wobbly smile. I ached to join in, but a sense of my own oddness would freeze me to the spot. Sometimes the pretending became too much and I sat on the hall steps and wept as the rest of the class was put through their paces at Scottish country dancing lessons. It must have been hellishly embarrassing for them. The janitor saw. He understood. His hands wobbled with regret when we chatted.

I adore dancing. I adore music and rhythms of all sorts. Music from all over the world is my friend, and as far I am concerned I cannot dance. Not really. I still can't make a fool of myself. In those days, there was no such thing as a guidance teacher, to whom I could apply for something else to do, something equally expressive, perhaps, and safely away from the music that tormented me; art maybe, as soothing therapy.

I am quite good at art and enjoy using an abundance of bright paints and pastels to make endless swirling patterns and shapes. Unfortunately, as I was unable to commit a likeness of a chair, a cabbage, or a pomegranate to the page, I was discouraged from following the art syllabus. It was decided early that I would be better off channeling my energies into more bookish studies. I knew that was a mistake: art would have been so good and healthy for me. Colors and the sweeping movement of brushes or crayons were always very soothing. With a bit of imaginative thought, I could have been allowed a seat at the back of any class to do my own thing. Instead, I was forced to don my skimpy gym clothes, sit to one side, watch and wait—again—while everyone else stepped around the hall, trying to pretend I was not there. What a waste of time and a howling humiliation that no one cared to deal with.

With a familiar dread, I understood that there were many other activities and sports I was expected to watch: running, tennis, hockey, badminton, golf, basketball. These activities, as well as several class outings, were denied to me because there was no use in my trying to join in. Team games, bonding, showers after a win or a loss? Not for me. I found myself asking, "What about me?" or "What should I do, Mrs. Sampson?" I dug these questions from my chest with a push of courage, though they often sounded uncomfortably plaintive. My enquiries put me at odds with a general expectation that I should stop drawing attention to myself. The shrugs and raised eyes of my classmates meant I eventually stopped asking and waited in a cold sweat to be overlooked.

The annual sports day was that singular, brilliant exception in a year of aching physical compromises: a fiesta at which everyone was buoyed up in the cheerfulness of the sun, the delightful prospect of the end of term almost within our grasp. Wide open fields gave me space to move without embarrassment and here I enjoyed running, knowing that the grassy sod cushioned my falls beautifully. I ran everywhere in the daylight and breezes, or I lay beneath cherry trees in bloom, smelling advancing summer in the wafting warmth.

Chapter Twenty-Two

When I was eleven, a second stay in the hospital was arranged to coincide with the summer holidays of 1976, so that I would not fall behind with any lessons. I missed the sun shining outside, but by then I was familiar with hospital routines, a veteran, so I settled in quickly. Veronica Youlton and I became best friends in Ward One. We broke the monotony with our game of let's pretend, "having lunch in a restaurant." Tasty food was ordered from a menu and we ate our meals seated on either side of her bed or mine. There was also a wonderful shop along the hospital corridor where the other children went. Every day they shared their sweets with me and sometimes when I was feeling bold, I would play long games of card poker with one particular girl using her minty "Matchmakers" candy sticks as the stake. I gobbled down my winnings before she could claim them back. She was very good-natured and offered me the box when she saw how much I liked them.

I understood more about my second operation, which was to stretch my hamstrings, an agonizing experience for which no previous pain prepared me. As the surgeon drew on me in several different colors, this time with great sweeping lines the length of my legs, I understood more clearly his intention, which was to help my legs to lie straighter and in a more relaxed position. He hoped this would be achieved by partially cutting the tendons at the back of the legs, across the top of my buttocks, then encasing my limbs in plaster from the top of the thigh to the ankle and leaving them to lengthen and settle for several weeks.

In recovery, I was largely confined to bed. I felt strangely dislocated, enfolded in unpredictable pain, as all around, the small rituals of normality continued, slightly warped from their usual pattern. Stitches, as well as heavy plaster casts, made it difficult to shuffle to the bathroom. Therefore, bed baths were the order of the day, tepid water applied with warm facecloths. I brushed my teeth over a plastic basin, carefully, so as not to splash the sheets, while pulses of pain fired through me like an unreliable electrical current.

After two weeks of lying in bed, my mother was asked to take me home and return with me to the hospital to have my plasters removed several weeks later. She was appalled at the prospect of carrying me at home in my heavy casts and protested that the arrangements she would have to make would be entirely unrealistic. She lived alone and the only bathroom in our house was up a steep flight of stairs. I was allowed to stay where I was, entirely unaware of the minor scandal my mother caused by refusing to cooperate with the hospital authorities. The nurse in charge soon exacted her revenge on me.

Over card games, books, magazines, and visits, each of us was dealing with our own pain. We also discovered friendships at our bedsides. The rest was killing idleness interspersed with bedpans for pissing and shitting in, overseen by nurses who watched carefully, lifted, wiped, and lowered.

When they found me slouching furtively on my pillows at a lopsided angle to avoid hurting, I was hoisted quickly under the arms by two nurses, so that I sat up straight, "One, Two—Three!" With sharp pains and shivering nerves I was left, hoping to feel less sore.

Endless petty cruelties were meted out to children at the mercy of a system that looked no further than the next procedure. And, though I met many angel nurses, I also encountered my share of sadistic bitches, one of whom—she just happened to be the ward matron— decided one day that it was "time those stitches came out." She prepared with a gleeful precision, pulling the curtain around my bed so that no one else could see how much she was going to enjoy this. Telling me to turn over on to my front, she snipped and then pulled every stained piece of thread out, one inch at a time. She scolded me as long spasms of pain convulsed my body and tears poured over my face. As instructed, I bit hard into the pillow while my bottom wept blood beneath her scissors. I sobbed and tried to stifle my screams and all the time, I knew: if it hurt so much, it was too soon.

Later I heard the other nurses whispering amongst themselves that yes, perhaps taking the stitches out had been premature and yes, it must have been bloody painful. A hasty remedy was found, though of course no one apologized. To the accompaniment of Demis Roussos' crooning voice comforting me over hospital radio, I spent mornings in the bath being urged not to squirm as a nurse poured libations of "artificial skin" into the tub, hoping that some would adhere to my backside and give it time to heal.

The day orderlies were cheerful, and lingered to talk as they cleaned and tidied the lockers and swept under the beds. My pal was a large, florid woman who seated herself beside me and in her soft Germanic vowels crooned to me, placing her big hands over my cheeks in a gesture of embrace. For that alone, I loved her. The night nurses had more time to spend at our bedsides. My special favorite would come and sit beside me. We would whisper for an hour together if I was lying wakeful, listening sadly to soft sounds of pain and loss on the ward. She didn't seem to think it odd that I so cherished her company. I have always been a cheap date, throwing my affections away on anyone who will show me the slightest kindness.

On the road to recovery, there were more visits to X-ray, "going to get your plasters off today!" and physiotherapy. Increasingly, my body felt like public property. Commands were issued by radiographers who lurked behind screens while I lay in panicked stillness beneath lowered radioactive panels. After a long wait of several weeks, technicians manhandled my limbs to cut away smelly plaster with fearfully sharp rotating blades, leaving thin, shivering, goose-bumpy legs exposed. My feet were pulled and pushed firmly by gentle physiotherapists with clear ideas of how far I should be able, by now, to inch myself along handle bars and how hard I should be working. How much? That was up to me, while they seemed to imply I should aim high. I was expected to walk to strengthen myself, to exercise, to learn, practice, to get better.

While I was in the hospital recuperating, my father came to see me, which was a rare treat. He was usually abroad during his postings, and it was his habit to visit Edinburgh over the winter holidays. While he was chatting to me, he quietly suggested that he could make all the necessary arrangements to send me to Switzerland. He explained that they could offer me special treatment there, massage, physical therapy, the works. They could fix me—if I would like that.

Father was trying to be helpful. I wondered, was this a competition between my parents? He seemed to overlook the fact that I was lying in a hospital where I had already been sent to "get better." Perhaps his suggestion was intended to complement my mother's ideas. I kept my face carefully blank.

The loss of privacy and personal space in which to grow in peace and make mistakes, this is what was missing in the hospital. Our free time was fitted uncomfortably around abrupt interruptions to make way for other people's requirements about which we knew very little: appointments which might or might not happen, and which brought boredom, shame, or pain in their unsteady wake. There was precious little room to let blossom the usual hopes of childhood and youth, or for peaceful enjoyment of personal pleasures. These were mostly shorn off and taken away with surplus body hair. Finally, I had no ambition left, except to get better and leave as soon as possible. If getting through all this was what it took, then I would do it.

As I left the hospital, I was given the back half of my plaster casts and asked to wear them every night, wrapped against my legs with bandages, supposedly to continue the progress with stretching. We did this for a few weeks until one morning I flung them into a closet. Some months later, they were discovered and thrown away.

Chapter Twenty-Three

Sometimes life was fun. At school we made several very sweet friendships. Father kept in touch with us in his long letters, which we read eagerly. In his words I could hear his voice, and his jokes made me laugh so hard that I was told off for unladylike behavior. We had nothing much to write in exchange, so we told him about our lessons and hoped that our end-of-term report cards would make him proud.

Martha liked to amuse me by playing the fool, especially in our home economics classes, which we generally agreed were a total waste of time. We lost interest in cooking after the boarding staff decreed that if in our morning lesson we made a portion of anything savory, we were to eat that instead of our usual set meal at lunchtime. In our first cooking class we were shown how to make toasted cheese. "Toasted cheese?" We looked on incredulously as cheddar was grated and carefully arranged on two dainty slices of bread, which were then cut into thin slices, stacked in a pyramid, and topped with a sprig of parsley. At home we had been toasting cheese sandwiches for years, with great homely slabs of bread and thick slices of Cheshire. We ate to fill our empty stomachs, not to waste time with polite exhibitions of dexterity.

I felt rather at sea in the sewing class, too. Being the only girl who proved unable to thread a sewing machine in front of the same fastidious teacher became the latest humiliation: *It's easy, Fran, see, you just go in round the back, through there like that, in this hole and under there* . . . It was futile, and dear kind Jane used to niftily thread it for me when teacher's back was turned. Often on the verge of bursting into tears, Martha cheered me up. She made me laugh helplessly by playing with a scrap of cloth: stuffed down her cleavage, round her throat as a choker, over her head as a hat, and all accompanied by suitably ridiculous expressions. I laughed so hard I almost collapsed. For the first time in my life I was sent out of a class and stood giggling in the corridor.

Our childhood diaries bear testament to our continuous obsession with food, for there was never enough to eat and we regularly filched slices of bread or packets of biscuits, which we would eat in the dormitory at night. "Today for breakfast we had . . . for lunch we had . . . it was rock-buns for tea and for supper it was . . ." Though food was in short supply and portions shrank as we grew older, I do remember one weekend when the cooks had catered for twenty-four girls and there were only twelve of us in the boarding house. I could not believe my luck when Martha tapped me on the shoulder. "Look!" she whispered. She had seen a whole tray of trifle left out on the trolley. That trifle was so delicious, just thinking of it makes my mouth water. Without saying a word to anyone, we ate steadily, consuming eight bowls of trifle each, before the house mistress realized what we were doing and crossly removed what remained, locking it in the staff fridge. It was the only time at school I was full after a meal.

I was forever being ticked off for unladylike behavior: refusing to wear my dressing gown and slippers, whistling, pelting along the downstairs corridor. Like the wind I ran, laughing. I didn't care tuppence for any reprimand. You could have threatened to expel me and I would not have stopped—that was probably the only joyful physical release I got. Running along dingy halls? Get a life, I hear you say . . . still it was something! Something I chose.

I knew what I wanted—I wanted to run, jump, move, sing, and make a lot of noise. I wanted to paint, make a wonderful mess, dance, rise up, and soar. I wanted to find my feet. More often than not, the communal arrangements we tolerated made that impossible. Impatience with my many confinements showed either in bold strokes of stubbornness, maverick failure to follow instructions, flaring temper and rudeness; or in their opposites: abject compliance, conformity, self-effacement, and silence. What a see-saw I worked, trying to find my balance.

Unable to take off and do my own thing, the school library became familiar to me as the place where I would be most likely to seek refuge from watching others laugh at games. I lost myself in historical novels and autobiographies of those famous people who had *done something interesting with their lives.*

In lessons, at arts, and on the sports field I was gently overshadowed by Martha, who was and is a superb all-rounder. I watched her talents unfolding, knowing that she was beautiful and deserved the best, helpless to stop the endless comparisons that ensued between us. Comparison is what schools do. I knew that she was more talented, more gifted than me, so when I won a prize—which I rarely did—I felt a fraud. Though that didn't stop me trying, there is something in the word "trying" that speaks of failure.

The good news is that I was too pleased by any academic success to resent it much in others, though of course I wanted to do as well as Martha and receive the praise that she did. I used to tease her. After an exam she would say, "I may look like I am overreacting, but *this time I know* I have fluffed that paper," and I would answer, "Of course you haven't, you have done better than me." I was always right, but at least she was safe from any real jealousy on that score.

Sometimes we made our own fun. I remember one weekend when the girls in the boarding house asked to go to the cinema, and not for a walk up Blackford Hill, which was the usual frog-march of deadly dullness on offer. We were told we could only go and see *Gregory's Girl* if it rained, so I declared, "Why don't we do a rain dance?" and we all trooped out to the garden and made a circle. Dramatically, in a loud voice, I asked for the rain to come, and we all sang and danced and clapped and cheered. The rain came. We went to the cinema.

As I grew older I was scolded that such games were frowned upon for young ladies, though I hardly cared. I was fending off loneliness that came with the realization that, as others went about their jolly business, I spent my days watching from the sidelines, scared to move, longing to join in. Scared to ask for a piece of cake when everyone else had one, because that would mean having to get up and walk across a room where special treats might be waiting, perched on a glass table top. If I missed my step and fell, the glass might shatter into thousands of pieces. The last thing I wanted was to cause a scene and it did not occur to me to ask for help. A lot of unwanted—and some faintly unwholesome—attention I received was so well-intentioned. Nowadays, I find it much easier to accept that most people are prompted to help by a loving impulse. As a pubescent girl, I could not feel the love, only the inquisitiveness, the opinions, and my crippling embarrassment, which gradually hardened into resentment as the years passed.

Without a murmur I was expected to subscribe to mediocre and limited expectations: no one noticed that it was mediocre and limited to expect me to do so much of nothing. Yet whole weeks were spent in a desert where color and vision were almost completely absent.

Chapter Twenty-Four

After the operation to lengthen my hamstrings, I was bequeathed continual spasms of pain in my legs, flares of agony, which came at any time without warning and leapt like licks of fire up my body. Nightmares kept me company for many months afterwards, whipping me out of sleep, rigid with panic, screaming. The girls in the dormitory were very understanding when I woke them. They didn't seem to mind, and soon dozed off again.

My left foot, in growing through the bone graft that had been installed years earlier, for a time became so painful that it could not bear any weight and I limped around, wishing I had something safe to lean on and worried that this new torture was going to last forever. No one knew what caused it or how to treat it and I was left to deal with the pain alone, fighting off the lingering suspicion of the boardinghouse staff that I was making it up to gain extra attention. Though why anyone would choose to take twenty minutes to cross an asphalt playground and whimper after each step simply to gain attention, is a mystery that was never solved. After a year or so, the pain disappeared as suddenly as it had come.

Invasive procedures, including a third operation at the age of sixteen, left scars over the lower half of my body; long, livid red lines that took years to fade. Incisions were sometimes so crudely repaired that decades later I could still count every stitch mark on my skin. Children giggled and pointed at these ugly lines whenever I used communal changing rooms and at the swimming pool. Soon, I hated going swimming, though it was one of the few activities that I could manage fairly well.

The agonized calculations inflicted on my small body by my well-meaning surgeon seemed to drive him into a frenzy approaching madness, so keen was he to try and "sort me out." I didn't understand what pain would follow from his consultations and didn't like to make a fuss. I had no real idea what anyone was talking about and wanted to avoid looking foolish, asking stupid questions. Most of the procedures for which my body was used as a medical playground were painful, pointless, and have since been discredited in favor of more holistic approaches to self-improvement and healing, based on movement and exercise.

Everyone in the world benefits from regular exercise. I have no doubt that if I stopped typing and took a firm decision to swim every day, my balance, coordination, and body strength would all greatly improve. However, the basic condition is underlying and non-progressive. I can write this now, though the constant exercises, operations, and bodily invasions have left their marks. The steel pin that my surgeon drilled into my right ankle joint—*how could he do that?*—permanently restricts the movement of that ankle, so that I trip more often, not less. Similarly, the partial cutting of my left Achilles tendon drops my foot so I often trip over it, my toes crumpling painfully as I hobble or fall. Arthritis, which riddles my joints—the right ankle in particular—is now only kept within manageable limits because I follow a fairly rigid diet to minimize flair-ups; and I wear a particular brand of very expensive footwear. I would not be able to walk without these shoes and count myself truly blessed that I can afford them.

By far, the worst effect of these intrusions into my dignity was the leadenness, the numbness that accepting such treatment forced into my mind and spirit. While still a young woman, my sense of adventure was hemorrhaging, following my blood down hospital drains. Logic and the dispassionate enquiries of those older and "better qualified" than me, rubbed away at what I knew about beauty, muting feelings of adventure that are usually invoked when we talk reverently of "Life!"

I may have received a great deal of attention, but it was not the carefree kind and seemed to come with a price tag: get better! People prodding and puzzling over me, cajoling with hopes and emotional blackmail wasted so much of my goodwill and precious time. My siblings probably resented the attention I received, and I resented their freedom. It became clearer to me with each passing day that nothing I did would pass without correction and nothing I said went without a comment, a puzzled look, a frown.

Singing was my salvation, as I sent out my voice to live for me. I read adventure and travel stories, and above all, I avoided attracting attention. I sat haunting the afternoon with my shadow.

My acquaintances occasionally comment on my ability to maintain deep quiet. They are impressed, unaware that I have mastered this skill because I felt forced to make a virtue of immobility. At an age when youngsters are hard wired to move and flit unceasingly, it was impossible for me not to want to do the same, no matter how clumsy I might have looked. But as I had no wish to attract attention to my "oddities" or be the subject of yet more speculation and insults, I forced myself to sit still. That I was often derided as "lazy" as a consequence is one of the many "no win" situations I learned to tolerate.

Chapter Twenty-Five

I spend my life living as if poised astride a fence, with one leg in the world of the "able bodied," the other inhabiting the world of the "disabled." Because I have never felt "disabled," when I was a child I believed that one glorious day I would get to do most of the ordinary things that you do.

Instead, growing up became a slow, heartbreaking awakening to the understanding that choices which others seemed to take for granted were forever destined to remain one tiny inch beyond my reach. Try as I might, I could not bridge the teasingly small gap that split me away from the carefree choices others took in their stride. To cope with my disappointment, I learned to adjust the brightness of my expectations so that they would not always blind me with tears: with piercing clarity I could understand your joy, though I felt unable to join it.

Although I am rediscovering much new happiness for myself, some things don't change. I still feel unable to take part with those who enjoy physical pursuits. I ache to be physical, though the world of the physically active does not comfortably cater to those who can manage some things, sometimes. The world of the physically active tends to be uncompromising.

After a long tussle with my feelings I may decide to tag along for the company and find myself forced to watch friends having fun while I simper from the sidelines, pretending that watching is the most riveting fun, that I really enjoy being the spare part in the party. Friends could easily slow down for me and opt not to go tree climbing or sky diving, but I hate speaking up, "Do you realize that I cannot walk as fast as you, and that I cannot shin up rocks?"

To avoid having to spell out my difficulties each time I am met with incomprehension, I often pretend that I have made a lifestyle choice, as it were, *not* to walk the mile, join a disco, and then walk home afterwards on a happy high. My most cheerful face is then called into service, as well as my usual apologetic explanation that I dislike dancing, when nothing is further from the truth.

If I can muster the strength, in among all the fun you are having, to explain that I would like a little help, I still feel like the solitary oddball at the party. Long, tall society may move smoothly, but it can be hellishly insensitive. Life doesn't mean to be unkind, it just is. I work so hard to fit in—and am successful so often—that when it would be helpful, no one notices I am disabled. The effort to be "just like everyone else" makes me break out in a sweat.

These days I am more resigned. I am beginning to recognize that love is all we need in order to see things clearly. My eyes are opened wide. I see: we are all disabled. Some of us by prejudice, some of us by fear, and some, by being misunderstood. We care so much what others think of us that our lives can become one long hobble to what we "should" or "should not" do next. None of us is truly "able bodied."

When I was about eight years old, I was sent off to enjoy a week's holiday at a camp for disabled children. To please my mother, I agreed to go, though I wanted to stay at home. I did not ask aloud, "Why are you sending me?"

I responded to the whole experience with a mixture of bravado and fear. For a week I was placed in with children who looked more "disabled" than me. I was confused. Gazing at contorted limbs and shaking wrists, I did not ask aloud, "Is this how you see me? Twisted and incoherent?"

Yet I discovered that, whatever their outward appearance, the "disabled" children I was roomed with at the holiday club were much kinder and more accepting than I was: friendly, well-adjusted, and gentle. Even so, I bullied them because I didn't want to be there. If this was how my family saw me, I was filled with shame. Despite that, I wanted to go home. I was in a trap.

Am I going to "get better"? No, I'm not. My condition is inoperable, permanent, and I am not "broken" in such a way that a tube of glue or a pile of nails will fix anything. Cerebral palsy or paralysis is caused by a lack of oxygen to the brain, usually because of suffocation at birth. Starved of oxygen, parts of the brain are damaged; in my case, those parts that have to do with coordination, balance, and the movement of the limbs. The outcome shows in differing degrees of spasticity, that is, tightness or loss of movement. "Spastic" is bandied around as an insult, but all it means is that certain muscles hold themselves in a spasm, while others are dead or have wasted away from lack of air or usage.

Since my last orthopedic operation, Mum has commented that she could have sanctioned more such operations to make me walk even better. She decided not to because she thought I had had enough. I don't think all the operations in the world would have offered lasting improvements to my gait. I found it alarming that my parents would even have considered allowing more pain for me, on the slim hope that doing so might make me more "normal." I could not believe that "walking like other people" mattered so much.

Chapter Twenty-Six

I come from a striving, ambitious family. I hardly wanted to be the singular letdown among us, so I decided early on that I *was not* going to be overlooked or written off. As the years passed, my failure to listen and inflexible attitude led me into many errors of judgment so that I lost too many years in a maze of wrong turns. Yet on a few rare occasions, my stubbornness has won me something precious. There was one battle I found myself fighting with Father which he would never win, one in which it didn't occur to me to admit defeat.

Between the school terms we often flew out to be with Father. We cantered away with our cases packed for warmer climes, eagerly anticipating the joys of flights unaccompanied: we freely played, giggled, and drank all the Coke and Fanta we desired, treated like royalty because of our diplomatic passports. Drunk on the freedom to be as greedy as we wished, Martha and I often drank twelve cans of Coke and Fanta, then worked our way through the Sprite and the 7UP until there were no soft drinks left. No wonder we were happy—the sugar high was fantastic.

We four children visited the country where Father was stationed, to stay for a month or so. He was often posted to countries where poverty was extreme and wars openly raged, or lurked smoldering just below the surface, hidden in the midst of lush green forests. Yet he seldom brought to our attention minor details such as civil war, unrest, or food shortages. By some miraculous contrivances and fancy footwork, the privileged children of Krisof Freyerling always had an abundance of food on their plates. I was grateful, without knowing the full extent of the difficulties Father must have faced every day. Only once in all the times we visited did he show his anger with our careless attitudes and even then, he spoke to us more in regret and sorrow.

I love my dad deeply. I can see in myself so much of him and understand that his flares of temper, though frightening, had more to do with his own fears than anything we might have done. Yet, in the years away from his oversight, as he travelled to places around the world for work and we all grew up at boarding schools, I was saddened that we drifted apart. Both our parents, in our absences from their homes, tended to forget that their children were growing, inching up into opinionated adulthood. They seemed to misread me, calling me lazy or complacent when I was just being an ordinary young girl, an adolescent resting.

During holidays with Father, there were occasions when our mutual sympathy faltered uneasily or split apart completely. Glimpses of uncomfortable memories catch me out at the oddest moments as I watch my own daughter growing up: a family skiing holiday in France during which I spent the days gazing hopelessly at families having fun on the slopes outside or luxuriating in well-earned *après ski*. With a regular supply of one-franc coins, I sat in the chilly coffee lounge and played on gaming machines. Some years later in Angola, there was a hot morning's riding on thin, high horses that were continually tormented by flies. Father kept "adjusting my stirrups" until I was perched lopsidedly, one leg dangling loosely and the other forced up almost to the top of the saddle. In despair at his inability to listen to me and sore with blistered ankles where my feet fell through the enormous stirrup irons, I slipped forward out of my seat and fell gently to the ground. I knew how to land safely as I had been riding ponies for many years by then. I awaited my latest telling off for letting the side down. Forbidden to explain my predicament, I was angry with him for the rest of the afternoon. I sat by the pool, nursed my blisters, and simmered.

One casualty of a fractured household is lost empathy, the kind of knowing that grows gradually through the intimacy of living together. People sharing the same space develop familiar rituals and recognize nuances in conversation and humor, all of which have to be politely explained to visitors so that we may make ourselves understood. Too young to excuse my father for not understanding me, his incomprehension took me by surprise and I withdrew.

Occasionally, readers have suggested that I skim too lightly over portraits of my parents and siblings. These are indeed sketchy at best, and people who have grown up with their family around them expect me to share more details about our daily lives: family jokes, catch phrases, a bit of Flemish dialect thrown in here and there for added flavor. Yes, I could perhaps ask my father to help out with that: Not only do I not speak Flemish, but I also don't know my birth family as well as I would like to. I love them and would willingly give all I have for them; even so, in addition to being preoccupied with my own struggles, ordinary details escaped me as we grew up living in different places, and it would be entirely unfair of me to invent them now. We did the best we could—all of us—but that does not mean that we were easy with each other.

Should I confess that, during school holidays in Edinburgh, Mum was usually absorbed with work, the fridge was often empty, and the four of us fought a great deal over nothing? We quarreled, continually either getting on each other's nerves or sinking into apathy. At least when we were with Father, the heat of the African tropics lifted our spirits. The intense light of morning pierced my usual lassitude and there was always time for swimming, for sunbathing, and for dancing at the evening functions. Accompanying all our usual activities, the swooping, elongated calls of large, flapping birds in the canopy woke us early and swung back and forth all day above our heads. Small geckos and lizards discovered in our rooms were a delightful reminder of wildness living nearby; and the ritual sipping of cups of smoky tea in the parched heat of late afternoon was infinitely consoling.

Father had developed a theory that it would be better for me to sit still. Yet, despite my frowning brow and my reluctance to be drawn into this conversation, he persisted, refining his belief that walking was bound to cause me pain and tax my body too far. Now he had a mission, urging me to take the weight off my feet, to rest on a soft seat, to be still and quiet. Feeling like an invalid under such treatment, I was typically resentful. His misplaced advice simmered and then his impatience boiled over when I was fourteen. My father made it clear that he wanted me to get a wheelchair. He insisted that my refusal to even think of using one was stupid, pubescent disobedience. For weeks, during one holiday in particular, I felt the full frown of his impatience when I flatly refused to consider any new confinement, even one with wheels. He lectured with quiet fury, "It will be easier! This will rest your joints, can't you see?" and when that failed to persuade me, he changed tack suggesting that, "It will be more relaxing—it will be fun for you!"

These reasons carry an echo of truth and are a touching reminder of how much my father would have liked more say in my choices. Using a wheelchair would have made my life more relaxing in many ways. My joints would be rested, and I would enjoy the freedom to move more quickly, in straight, solid, respectable lines. I would not look too out of place in a social gathering; I would just be shorter than everyone else, so there would be lots of stooping and looking down at me.

My father saw in my closed, angry face the look of his stubborn wife. Yet nothing indicated more clearly how little he understood me, now that I was growing and cherishing opinions of my own. I don't blame him, as he clearly didn't get much opportunity to be with this girl of his, who had taught herself to walk at a hobble and run fast while living so far away from him. Where there was once a sweet fondness, now we felt mutual hostility. He simply did not realize that I enjoyed walking. I loved my small freedoms and it was my choice to move myself by myself.

"Assistance" in the form of a hand up, an arm to lean on, or a wheelchair, is only ever welcome when it is chosen. It made me bristle that he expected me to play pathetic when what I most desired was to *fall and learn the power of getting myself up again to have another go.* The next time I might get it right. The challenge was what I most enjoyed.

In any case, nowhere was the real reason for my father's insistence made plain: he, like my mother, was deeply embarrassed by the way I looked when I walked unaided. They both shrank inwardly while watching me dance, though, understandably, neither would admit their distaste. Instead, I was cast as the family nuisance, disobedient, and much too obstinate for my own good.

The rest of the family seemed equally baffled at my insistence on being independent. There was much loving "protection" extended to me; and in exchange for all their help, I was expected to listen to varying opinions and agree with them. Above all, I had to do what was expected of me. "We only want what is best for you," was a refrain I got used to hearing.

How difficult my parents have found it to love me as I am, regardless of the opinions of others. My awkwardness seems to have been something of a crucifixion for them. Little wonder, then, that I found it ever harder to love myself. Children are only copy machines, after all. During the shaky teen years in which I started to stretch, measure, and calculate for my independence, I understood that for once I must be true to myself. I *could* run, I *could* jump, I *could* take myself where I chose to go. So I had no hesitation in being cast as an irritating pain in the backside who walked. For me to subscribe to a belief that I was embarrassing *because I walked differently* would have been the end. Why should I surrender my freedoms?

Years later, I had an interesting conversation with Martha. She was training to be a doctor and was at an advanced stage in her studies.

Her class of students had been exposed to questions of social pressure around disability and she was learning anew, through watching films and interviews of those affected, how hard it is to resist the expectations of others once a child with mobility difficulties grows beyond a "cute and cuddly" age. She remarked, her voice rising incredulously, "A lot of adults get wheelchairs when they can walk perfectly well; it's just that their families find it all too embarrassing!" She was shocked. Before her insight dawned, she had not seen behind my scowling face or my snappy, "No thank you, I can manage!" to the reasons for my hostility and resentment.

When anyone succumbs to social expectations to use a wheelchair, their bodies become more sedentary than ever and their muscles slide into atrophy, making the chances for mobility even more remote. While "able bodied" adults are given extensive rehabilitation to allow them to walk after accidents and strokes, those born with a physical impairment that affects their mobility seem to receive less encouragement. Why is that?

I am doubly fortunate that my mother trained in medicine. Without her prior knowledge, would she have been able to withstand the pressure of pitifully low expectations for me? How many others with issues like mine are languishing in the shadows of institutional ignorance because their families listen politely to advice which owes more to prejudice and speculation than to hard facts or compassion? If it wasn't for my mother's decision so often to disagree, to go it alone, I would be in a "home," possibly dead, having led only a teeny little bit of a life. No one would have known anything about me, or uncovered the thoughts lurking behind my eyes. The smallness of my life would have remained a hidden loss, overlooked, as the lives of so many disabled adults are overlooked.

It is one of my particular flaws that I delight in proving people wrong, especially any hapless professional wearing a white coat who strays into the path of my determination: the child psychiatrist who offered her professional opinion that, "She will not amount to much";

my innocent friend at school who confessed that her father, another expert with dozens of letters after his name, had said, "Fran will be in a wheelchair by the age of forty." The difficulty was to decide who might be right and who was just an ignorant twit.

The general and widespread ignorance I came up against made me a hostile woman, abnormally resistant to advice and unable to select out those thoughts that I might have found useful. Instead, time and again, my expectation was confirmed that no one understood me— how isolating that is.

I was not the only member of my birth family to endure some hard knocks, but now I have decided that the only thing to do with suffering is to find some way to turn it to good account, so that it does not defeat you. The only thing to do with tears is water your flowers with them, so that there is something to show the world when the sun comes out. The only use for anger is to let it propel you towards activities that renew your hope and joy, or towards those you love. And to love yourself despite everything, that is The Big Idea.

Chapter Twenty-Seven

While I was promoted to prefect in fifth year—a job I hated—Martha, who had done so much to merit recognition, was passed over. After that, I knew school was a sham and I was happy when Martha started going to a much larger school where she could give full expression to her talents. There she thrived, while living at home for fifth and sixth year. I was asked if I wanted to go too, but I refused, certain that Martha did not need me dogging her steps. I stayed where I was, boarding and more alone than ever, trapped in my fantasies of action, of love; and yearning to discover where I might fit.

Still doing what I was told, and with every minute of my day programmed in advance, I had become a studious, rigid, and depressed pupil, increasingly silent and sullen. I took refuge from my unhappiness in studying because that was better than contemplating the hole that was growing inside me, the hollow shell I was becoming, and which I cloaked beneath biting humor or feigned indifference.

I was able to take something positive from most of my studies, but not math. That was a constant torment and tease; like being forced to watch the beautiful young man you adore who doesn't see you, no matter how often you prance near him in a sparkling spandex suit. No one understood why I could not get my head around it, and I could not understand why no one understood that I could not understand it. I am sure there must be a club for those of us who are perfectly capable and intelligent, but for whom math is a foreign language.

How I wish that someone had seen that my confusion was not a sign of terminal stupidity and said to me, "It's all right, Fran, you can just give this up now. You never have to see a quadrilateral equation again." I would have cried with relief. Instead, I wasted many hours wrestling with my version of hell, which was one reason my other grades failed to hit the stellar heights of those achieved by my siblings. No one troubled me with physics or chemistry.

Instead, I played games with the fluency of languages. To my surprise, I discovered that I excelled at practical criticism in French—not much use, admittedly, when facing questions in the dole queue, but still, we all have to start somewhere. I found it easy to pretend I was someone else and discovered an ability to soar away in my imagination with any character in a book willing to come with me. At last, I received some genuine praise from an otherwise hectoring and puzzled tutor. To my young, jaundiced eye, she wore too much lipstick and her lips pouted in a scowl while she lamented the inconsistencies of my approach: "If the cap fits, wear it!" she repeated often, advice which I found baffling, though I did not ask, "What do you mean?" and never discovered what translation and caps might have in common.

When I was allowed to express myself, I did well enough even by my perfectionist standards, so English was my favorite subject. I liked geography because it was often about other people, living somewhere warm, or in places cold and wild, with the wind in their faces. I adored Mrs. Bethany. Funny, tolerant, and approachable, in her classes I made a point of sitting in the front seat so that I could feel the happiness and strength radiating from her. She, in her quiet way, kept me going during my shaky middle years. She was so *normal*. She never once commented or asked me rude questions, and she knew that I hid a sense of humor under my prickles.

I was young when I encountered my first existential crisis. I was on a family holiday, gazing in from behind a barbed-wire fence at an animal park enclosure and absently fondling the head of some passing goat, my wrist turned sideways to reach its silky ears. Aged ten, standing in sawdust amidst the smells of animal dung, I realized that one day I would grow up, and I would be expected to earn my keep: But how? The question of what I was going to do with my life started its long spooky dance with me. How was I to earn a living if I couldn't opt for casual employment, nor be a doctor, had only sporadic success with the sciences, was useless at math, and deeply shy?

My second identity crisis came to haunt me some years later and started when I was clambering up to class after morning assembly. It was a Wednesday and I was in fourth year of secondary school, so I would have just turned sixteen. As I ascended the stairs, my eyes alighted on the portraits of all the past head girls of the school, their proud pictures pinned to the wall of the stairwell. The years had rolled by seamlessly; each year the line of smiling, youthful faces grew longer. There was a space ready and waiting for a portrait of this year's star pupil. The evidence thus laid out before me of the passing of time abruptly convinced me that any dreams I might cherish of "getting better" were deluded. If, after all these years and all the well-meaning efforts played out on my body I was still disabled, I always would be.

This hammer blow to my happiness winded me so that I barely crept into the classroom before I rested my head on my desk and wept. Thankfully, the break after morning assembly was noisy so I did not attract much attention. The day pupil I usually sat alongside listened sympathetically to my stammering excuses. She did not try to jolly me along. She was simply quiet and kind and I was profoundly grateful. Her understanding was enough to get me through the rest of the day, until I reached the cover of darkness and my bed. I spent that night wondering what would become of me.

It is hard to find peace or privacy anywhere in a boarding house. On the one hand, this kept me from sinking in sorrow. On the other hand, I felt clogged up and artificial, and there was really nowhere to take these feelings to release them. I swallowed them down into my already aching body and just got on with each day. The mechanics of that were easy enough. We were not expected to think too hard for ourselves. Everything was planned for us, so it was fairly simple to live on autopilot.

When I had moments to reflect, some things were certain in my naive, unhappy mind. I would have to abandon all my dreams, any pictures in which I could still dimly see myself smiling, gaily singing, pirouetting, and waltzing through my days. Growing up wasn't going to be easy or fun, after all! I could see that I would have to get a desk job, and by now I was so full of groveling that almost any desk would do. That was all I could see in my future: a huge, brown desk with piles of paper on it, behind which I hid each day, filing away other peoples' lives. There was sure to be lots of sitting.

The truth which I conceal uneasily behind my compliant exterior is that I am a naturally active woman. Given half a chance I can also be gregarious and giggly. Yet, by the age of ten, I was already worrying what I would do when I grew up and had to make enough money to keep myself warm and fed. In the growing-up years, when adults think their children are carefree, laughing and running, dancing and playing the fool, I became ever more preoccupied. I pushed my worries aside, though the question, "What am I going to do?" hung low over my head: Where would I go without the school gates to protect me? What would I live on?

I cannot understand why no one else showed the slightest concern about my career. Perhaps I am wrong. Perhaps everyone was very concerned, though they hid their worrying well. I don't remember my parents raising the subject of money, or reassuring me that I would not end up destitute, living alone, and hungry in an attic. Was it evident that I would only have a small, confined life, dependent on family largesse or state handouts? Or was I simply so anxious that I wasn't listening? Certainly no one expected me to meet, even less marry, a Prince Charming who could keep me in the lap of luxury. Did my family see me living the single life, bent over a table in a basement doing filing? Maybe they thought I had some great and glorious future in mind.

Perhaps that is one thing boarding school does badly: it distances its children from ordinary people they might get to know, who could offer support when faced with life's choices. Ordinary, gentle people would have seen nothing wrong in studying for enjoyment and might even have encouraged me to take up English literature, languages, Sanskrit, art history, whatever I felt like. They would not have written me off had I chosen a "soft" option. I might even have had some fun!

I eventually made up my mind to study law. I had no real idea what this meant, though it sounded grand, and that appealed to me; in any case, I had gained qualifications adequate to offer the choice of going North or West. I smiled, as I was sure to be guaranteed some respect. No one could accuse me of laziness or lack of talent now; nor would anyone assume I was mentally challenged. It also became necessary to escape the suggestions of my mother's well-meaning friends that they might be able to find me a nice small job somewhere in the corner of an office, shuffling bits of paper.

Chapter Twenty-Eight

I had no way of knowing that, if I searched the world over for a painful vocation which would bring out the worst in me, I could hardly have chosen better than law. In retrospect, I can cut myself some slack. I urgently needed to establish my credentials as an ordinary, intelligent woman, by studying something heavy. Unfortunately, I cannot carry a sign on my back which says, "I have a legal degree—please don't treat me like an idiot!" and now I accept that an expensive education makes little difference: I still encounter people on the buses and in the street who talk at me as if I am hard of hearing and one penny short of a pound. I might have known that I cannot single-handedly shift the prejudices of an entire population.

Having been ceremoniously dumped outside the gates of Aberdeen University, my future seemed anything but bright; I was terrified. I was eighteen and a late developer. I could easily have passed for fourteen. For many years I had worn my hair long, but squashed out of sight in an unflattering bun pinned to the back of my head, like a Victorian school teacher. Latterly, Mum cut my hair into a short bob.

In an effort to smarten up our ideas before we left, the school organized a few dances to which boys were invited, though with typical self-effacement, I placed myself behind the drinks table, at the serving hatch, or kitchen sink so that I rarely had to confront my oddness in mixed company. I shied away from situations where I might meet with unfavorable comparisons. What a pity I didn't realize that not every boy was as mixed up and judgmental as I was. One youth at our annual school dance, I think his name was Chris, even asked me to dance and was sweetly persistent. I was cringingly shy and incredulous and he gave up asking after twenty times, though he kept glancing in my direction. I had never been kissed, though I longed to be. Admittedly, my options as a schoolgirl were limited. Nor did I have the inclination or energy to hang around outside the army barracks up the road, or invite any man to shin up and down the drainpipes outside the dormitory, as one of my classmates arranged.

My best pals were friendly girls, sweet and kind; the teachers I had were amusing and much of my schoolwork was interesting. Yet I knew that I was hiding, and my favorite hiding place was between the covers of my latest book. Looking back through my sister's collection of photos, in many casual poses I am clutching a volume. For years, I got my kicks by reading. Sadly, reading is often an up-market version of voyeurism rather like television: I read about what others were doing, while all I was doing was reading. I was probably addicted, using books to avoid facing uncomfortable realities and hide from all kinds of pain. Whenever I felt at a loss, which was most of the time, I reached for my latest paperback. No one thought this was a bad idea. Mum said, "If you can't do it, you can at least read about it."

By the age of fifteen, the only person who had fondled me was an older man on a transatlantic flight so full of himself that he thought his wife could not see that his fingers were teasing the breasts of the girl seated next to him. Of course she could, and watched the whole performance with a fleeting smile of resignation as I helplessly tried to get away. At five in the morning, with most sensible people asleep and no spare seats anywhere, I endured his heavily cologned hands running all over me because I didn't want to cause a fuss.

He may have enjoyed himself but I was morbidly self-conscious. I hated my body. I hated walking, I hated sitting still. I squirmed in the realization that in my able-bodied sisters and among all my friends, there was inevitably someone preferable to choose from. Some years earlier, Elouise had blazed a trail to Aberdeen University where Martha and I followed. "Ah, so you are Elouise's sister!" became a routine reaction wherever I was introduced, as boys' glances slid sideways over my shoulder, into someone else's gaze.

A wry smile may surface now, but I would like twenty years of my life back. From the first moment I found myself seated in the uncomfortable and rare confines of the law library as a student trying to make sense of legal rubric (*God on earth—what is this?*), I knew that my brain was really not enjoying what I was forcing it to do. Yet something in me refused to admit defeat. I just couldn't bring myself to throw it all away, transfer into a general arts degree, or go home with my tail between my legs. If I gave up, I would have to take that job in filing, after all. No, thank you: I decided to finish my studies. I opted for the age-old strategy called "wait and see."

While Elouise continued her academic studies at Aberdeen and kept a benign eye on her sisters, Simon was studying at York University, playing games with a relatively new invention, computers. He had found his passion and spent many days working in his room. Even so, during the holidays whenever he had occasion to cook a meal or when we were together, he must have noticed my habitually gloomy expression. He enthused over my writing and took time to suggest other avenues for me to explore. His faith in my talents has always been in the background, sustaining me.

Inside, I carried a sinking feeling, which reminded me constantly that, for the most part, legal studies and I were not a match made in heaven: I was a round peg in a firm and unyielding square hole. Predictably, I did well in theoretical subjects like legal philosophy or ancient Chinese law, where my imagination found space to move. If I could have been gentle with myself, I might have chosen more subjects such as legal history, which offered genuine enjoyment. Instead, I deliberately chose subjects for which I had less aptitude, believing that, since they were difficult, they were more worthwhile. Nor was I calculating enough to appreciate that if I enjoyed what I was studying, I would probably achieve a better final grade, and no one in the world would have cared a monkey's chuff whether I had done legal history or criminal procedure to get it. In so many ways, I have been my own worst enemy. But then, I worried about things that other people seemed to skim lightly over on their way to a better time.

We had entertaining lecturers, bright gems who lit up the room with their sardonic humor and love for their subject; people it was a pleasure to learn from, and whom I came to admire and respect. They were funny and thoughtful. Probably bored spelling out the same lectures over and over, they did not communicate that to us. Instead, they reminded us repeatedly that we were the cream of the crop, so to speak, which made us feel terrific. I enjoyed legal theory, but in the learning of law and procedure I knew that I was only using one part of my brain. I was going to have to admit that creativity mattered to me, but not yet. I still believed in suffering and martyrdom.

Chapter Twenty-Nine

There was freedom on campus, as well as peace to study as hard as I wanted without being written off as a total swot. That made a welcome change from school. In some ways, I was lucky. Unlike my mates, I did not go through agonies of homesickness. I had been severing ties with home for many years and felt faintly scornful of grown women weeping as they bid their loving parents goodbye.

I made some wonderful friends in halls of residence. My neighbors, all girls, were kind and full of laughs. Occasionally they would persuade me to go out for a drink and I would get easily and delightfully sloshed. Dragged home between two strong sets of shoulders, I could hardly put one foot before the other, and was in hysterics all the way. I was, and still am, a very happy, giggly drunk. I was in heaven as one of the crowd, being liked enough to share the laughs. Susan even removed my socks and shoes before tipping me into bed, and I could hardly believe that this cheerful, smiling soul did not recoil in disgust at the sight of my mutilated feet. I adored her because she was accepting and tactful.

Hall routines felt familiar: I was used to eating adequate meals in large cafeterias. I began noticing that when any young handsome man offered to help carry my meal tray to a table, he invariably hailed from Louisiana or Georgia and was hoping to use breakfast as a heaven-sent opportunity to convert me to his brand of religion. I was frequently assisted to my seat and then earnestly lectured about the love of Christ for sinners. Over tea and toast, I was told that I was going straight to hell, mostly because I had the temerity to disagree with them. Sincere gentle women, too, would gaze earnestly at me, hoping that their fervor would persuade me to join the crusade. If they had understood I was unfazed by what they told me, they could have saved themselves a great deal of trouble: In so many ways, I was already in hell and a little more would hardly be noticed. At the time, I could pass myself off as a cynical atheist, though anyone caring to look below the surface would have seen my despair.

In matters of the heart, I could not help noticing that I seemed to attract into my orbit men with low ambitions: the aged janitor with bright blue eyes and a charming smile who offered me a sweet as an inducement from his pocket; the older man with a bad marriage; the callow youth on a crusade. I was sufficiently aware to suspect that unless I raised my game, until I could care for myself, I was not going to catch the dream. It has taken me many years to realize that low expectations give poor results. Another fifteen years would pass before I stopped, listened, and started experimenting to find ways to turn my life around.

In the meantime you may ask, were there no dates, no kisses, no frantic groping sessions after dances? There were not. I enjoyed discos where the forgiving dimness sent me spinning in a frenzy of delight. I sang along to the frenetic music and rhythms of Michael Jackson, so much better than those soppy New Age Romantics who wailed out of tune and could not hit the high notes. I danced until I fell over and then got up and skidded some more. In the darkness, who cared what I looked like? I happily danced by myself. If any man had been brave and joined me, I am sure I would have smiled at him, though I was much too complicated for anyone wanting a fun date. There were no embraces from gentle escorts at the end of the evening.

Did I wear nice clothes, pretty dresses, or strappy sandals? Not often, since I felt ill at ease in flimsy clothing and found it strange to wear skimpy tops, slinky skirts, or any footwear with a heel. Slender courts that match pretty clothes are simply impossible—and I love shoes. Anything except "A-line" skirts let down to a modest length, sensible shirts tucked in at the back, and boring flats were not really an option. How does a girl dress elegantly when all she possesses are scuffed trainers and black lace-ups? With my boyish figure I felt ridiculously self-conscious, like the stick of celery at a luxurious buffet. Did I wear makeup or perfume? Once or twice, in a cack-handed way, but then, no one shared with me the mysteries of pretty women, so I was self-taught, though I have little natural talent for self-decoration.

Do I remember parties? Yes, occasionally. Memories of one particular evening have stayed with me and still make me grin. A crowd of us in halls was invited to someone's room where the drink was flowing. Though I seldom drank, that evening I got very merry and laughed for hours, sitting on the floor with my back to the wall. That was a great party because there was absolutely no room to dance so no one needed even to think of asking. Perfect! We just sang along to the music. I didn't have to stand either except to stagger off to my room at the end. By then, everyone else was staggering too, so for once I didn't feel out of it. Sad, in a way, to remember one solitary piss-up, but it was fabulous!

I played the usual games of catch up, to get to lectures on time, trying not to skid and fall on wide slabs of stone. Out on the streets I was self-conscious, while I pretended to laugh gamely, as if it was my choice to be the odd one out. Having a physical handicap was seen as rather eccentric: "I think I will just go and get some CP for a while, why not? It broadens the mind to experiment occasionally with different lifestyle choices." People walked past me as if I wasn't there, continuing their conversations over my head: invisible Fran. I know now that I wasn't the only lonely one. There were others who felt isolated. Young adults are typically very constrained by their need to belong and be taken seriously. It is a rare youngster who does not care what others think of them, though I can bring to mind one or two—I remember them because they were unaffected and friendly towards me. If I had taken risks in conversation, I might have made deeper friendships among those I had something in common with, even if our sense of kinship had its origins in feelings of isolation. In student halls, I attracted those others with broken limbs. Seeing the parade we made, Elouise commented dryly, "Perhaps you should diversify a bit." Hey, it wasn't entirely my choice you realize. To the smooth-limbed athletic variety of lawyer I was a bit of an embarrassment.

By slow degrees, as I got my bearings, I noticed that I enjoyed the company of men, so long as it was understood that they were not interested in me in "that" kind of way. I became outrageously flirtatious and we had some good laughs. Where was the harm in that? I was never in the frame for anything more serious. Though I put on a good show in happy company, I was afloat in a churn of doubts. I sat with my workbooks, worried about my future and kept largely to myself.

Many years later I met one of my classmates unexpectedly in a department store. He shifted uncomfortably and one of the first things he said was, "I'm married now!" to stave off my smile, as if he thought I might start kissing him right there among the china and lampshades. I don't think it occurred to him that I might be married, too.

Chapter Thirty

Getting hitched was the last thing on my mind at that time, and there wasn't exactly a queue of eligible chaps lusting to take out or take on a silent, mournful woman with severe hair, even if she was rather beautiful in a strange sort of way. What was she thinking? No idea. I was all at sea in my unhappiness. Unsurprisingly, I was not seen as a sexy woman, more as someone who might appreciate the odd act of charity now and then, when no one else was looking.

As a teenager, I said to my mother, "I am never going to get married." I had been hoping that maybe, just maybe, we might have a talk. I was really hoping to pick up some tips about sex—for me I mean. Maybe she misunderstood. All she answered was, "Oh, good!" I was at first taken aback and then disappointed that Mum so easily cast me in the role of spinster. At the time we simply didn't have the kind of relaxed relationship that made intimate conversations a possibility.

One thing I knew about sex, with desperate certainty, is that if I was lucky enough to get any, becoming pregnant was out of the question. For me, that would have been a disaster straight out of a Dickens novel. I knew that once could get a girl "into trouble." The way I felt about fate, I knew that I would be the unlucky one. I doubted that Mum would have been very understanding, somehow. Assuming I didn't have an abortion, social workers would have been all over me, urging me to have my child adopted as, "clearly you are unable to manage." It may sound harsh, old-fashioned, and improbable, but every skeptic who had been watching, waiting for me to fall flat on my face would now have seized their chance to whisper with pained satisfaction, "You see? I told you she couldn't manage!" I'd never have heard the end of my "irresponsibility." I felt the eyes of the world on me.

I don't think my fears were much exaggerated. There is a parallel universe that many disabled adults live within. It feels like one of the last great taboos of growing up with a physical handicap: Sex for spastics? How would they cope? We have no idea, so we will just leave them to work it out for themselves. How many disabled single mothers do we see in our towns and cities? You may say I am being too dramatic. You may wish to hasten to my side to reassure me that no, it wouldn't have been like that. But I was not going to risk finding out. This wasn't the kind of research I was used to, though I knew that the omens were not promising and I didn't fancy existing alone in a studio apartment.

I was so terrified of ending up pregnant that I clung to a chemical contraceptive for over twelve years, and in every way my loyalty was bleak and unrewarding. Sex was as rare as a swallow flying over the roost in February, but, ever in search of that miracle, I clung to The Pill although using it made me fat, square, lumpish, and deeply depressed. It wasn't until I decided that I had finally had enough, threw my "Pregonon" in the bin, and fifteen pounds of weight dropped off me, that I suddenly felt lighter, like I might laugh sometime soon, without the aid of alcohol to lift my inhibitions. It only took me twelve years to realize. I like to look on the bright side—at least I didn't fall pregnant before I met Mr. Right.

I met Mr. Wrong several times, although sex, as in full sex, was forever elusive. One young chap liked to imply that he took pity on me, really. He spoke in confidential tones to Martha about my shortcomings. Once, they went for a long walk and when Martha returned she said, "I don't know why you are with him!" I wasn't for much longer. Another chap was a mixed bundle of insecurities himself and disliked me for my snobbish upbringing. He wished I didn't look so foreign—what could I have done about that, exactly?

I know, if anyone had said that to you, you would have ended your friendship there and then; but I spent many years feeling so pathetically grateful for any attention, particularly any sexual interest, that I only ended these relationships when the truth was right up in my face shouting, HAVE SOME SELF-RESPECT, FOR CHRIST'S SAKE! Once, when a friend of my lover told him he thought it was disgusting he was "shagging a cripple," a part of me wished I could have been very grown up. Instead of reacting with shock and retreating further into my solitary unhappiness, I wished I could laugh it off, as my lover clearly hoped I would. He grinned at such foolishness, but I might as well have been condemned. I wished that particular ignoramus and I could have broken out the coffee and biscuits and had a full and frank discussion about exactly what shagging meant, for me and my lover. Or rather, what it didn't mean. "Sex" was either making out with petting thrown in as an afterthought or a frantic, interrupted grope that came to nothing. I like sex, as most women do, so my partner and I usually salvaged quite a lot of pleasure from our experiences together, in the myriad ways that one can without actually doing the deed. My then lover was good in bed: patient, thoughtful, kind, and amusing. He enjoyed holding me down and watching emotions flit over my face: the delight, the joy, and despair in my eyes as I came fiercely to a climax and then wept with emotion. Did we have the delight of full, warm, sexy sex? No. That did not feature during my time at university.

It has always been difficult for me to make love, so natural spontaneity takes a battering. I do not move easily or comfortably in bed. I am a bit clumsy, with knees and elbows that dig into soft places where it hurts—a big turn-off. My legs refuse to do what I hope they will; alas, my hips are narrow and my thighs are fixed half-shut. Making love is hard work and often painful.

Surveys teasingly reveal that most couples who have been together for many years are happier sharing a cup of tea than having sex. With that politeness, which feels so frightfully British, we pretend to be scandalized and change the subject. And me? I would have loved a "normal" sex life, though in retrospect I am not sure there is any such thing. Although I dreaded pregnancy, I also harbored a fear of what might *not* happen if any man was interested to take things further. Both fears were equally tenacious and made me distance myself from serious attachments. Rather than explore this dilemma in a loving way with any young man brave enough to care, I opted out by default, not because I chose to. Others may have held hurtful or outrageous opinions about me, but I did not have the words or the confidence to confront them. If love had found me, things might have turned out differently. In the meantime, I told no one the truth. I looked after myself as best I could and kept quiet, though I was ashamed.

These days, I doubt that having a healthy sexual appetite was something I needed to be ashamed of. It was not something scandalous that I chose out of a box, after all. Like my big hands or my short-sighted eyes, my sex drive is just one of the gifts handed to me for life. What was I to do with my raging frustration? I regularly spent evenings masturbating, having marathon sessions in which I pushed myself as hard as I could and counted thirty-one or thirty-two orgasms. Surreal and amazing, it was also lonely, hardly something I could talk about with my friends—"Oh, Edith, you'll never guess what I was doing last night!" I was numb for days afterwards but at least the disbelief that washed over me was the outcome of something tangible. And sometimes, I could not help being pleased with myself.

Chapter Thirty-One

I found work as a legal trainee after I had received well over one hundred letters of rejection. After the first hundred or so, I stopped counting. I could not decide whether to mention my disability in my application—if I didn't, I risked being accused of dishonesty and shown the door; when I did, my application was usually thrown in the bin.

Eventually, I learned what works at interview: Take a taxi if it is raining, otherwise you will leave a wet seat behind you and won't get the job. Don't grovel. When someone asks, "So, what is the hardest thing for you about having a disability?" be amusing. For God's sake, make them laugh! It was my mother who suggested I might try my luck with, "Finding shoes that I can walk in!" which cheered up the atmosphere nicely. Everyone was expecting me to come out with a sob story; instead, I was admitting that my shoes tended to be boring. With this line I did almost secure a job in an excellent firm that recognized my potential, though by that stage, rather late in the day, I was too fearful to await the outcome of their plodding selection process. I have also since discovered that, had I waited a little longer, I might have secured work with the local council, which would have ensured me an excellent training. I had so little faith in myself, I was like a dog searching for scraps under the table—I missed the meal that was laid out for me above.

Indeed, I ended up with scraps. I was in a job that felt like the end of the world. It looked respectable and ordinary from the outside, housed as we were in a genteel Victorian building in the west end of Aberdeen; but I was very isolated in a small, shabby practice. Even before I started work, nothing could persuade me that I liked the look of the dark brown ceilings and the threadbare carpets.

There was the boss whose office was downstairs; there was his darling protégé whose office was opposite; and there was me, upstairs in my room under the attic. There was also a newly qualified assistant, a kind woman who, predictably, was expected to take me under her wing. She was briefed to provide nurture for me, while the men, vastly superior, were not expected to involve themselves much with my progress. After the first introductions were dispensed with and after my first few mistakes—which all trainees were bound to make—they left me entirely alone, no doubt hoping that one day I would just stop coming into the office and they would not have to pay me a pittance for doing nothing.

No one gave me any work. I read the entire "Poldark" series from beginning to end. I came in late. In a stupor of exhausted neglect, I tried to pretend I was doing research by reading old files and absorbing from them the language and conventions of legal correspondence and commerce.

I finally found something to do in the cash room compiling a debt collection account; but as I had little ease with figures, this too proved to be a slow, crushing disappointment. Every time the compilation of the quarterly account came around, dear Patricia approached me with a doom-laden expression—we both knew that she would have to spend precious time unpicking my compilation to find the one mistake I had made. When I saw her approaching, I wanted to run screaming in the opposite direction. Instead, I grimly accepted my next challenge and hoped that this time I might be rewarded with a perfect column of figures. Not once did it come out right, and Patricia's expression grew grimmer by the quarter.

By some miracle of lateral thinking, she and I hit on debt collection, which I enjoyed very much. Chasing debtors by telephone with a smile of steel and a deep determination in my voice seemed to work well, and I enjoyed the game. I knew it was a game. Why else would we be spending twenty pounds, say, chasing a debt of £7.50? "Because of the principle!" admonished Patricia, who smiled happily now that we were successful coconspirators. I admired the gentlemen on the other end of the telephone who told me for the twentieth time that "the check is in the mail." We had a good laugh. I learned something about how a cash room works, about compiling court papers, and pursuing debts in court.

Finally, for the last six months of my two-year contract, in a blaze of glory I got some real work to do, when my boss tied his firm with another and there was help extended to me by a wonderful assistant who taught me something, for a change. They could not discharge me if they had not shown me anything, and a sense of shame came galloping to my rescue.

I sharpened up. I hardened my stance and sent out a good CV. I am fond of telling my friends that in one day I received three job offers and a proposal of marriage. When the partners saw me leaving, they asked me to stay and, in utter astonishment at their request, I refused outright, "No! Thank you!" Clutching my letters of discharge, I was on my way out the door.

And the marriage proposal? That was only a charming drunkard I happened to bump into on the way to the station, after the second successful job interview of the day. He had a beautiful mop of golden hair and the bluest eyes I ever did see. He was lounging good-naturedly with his father, catching the rays of a weak midday sun, already firmly in the grip of his cups. He muttered, "Marry me, dear? Make a man happy!" and I smiled and said "No, thank you."

Chapter Thirty-Two

Once I got the hang of it, I enjoyed my first real job, based in Edinburgh. I had moved back home with Mum for a while. Poor Mum, I was always popping up like a bad penny. On the plus side, I managed to pass my driving test at the fifth attempt and felt very grown up. Here was an achievement we were all proud of. To celebrate, Mum bought me a red, second-hand Mini in which I set off to work each morning, pulling out the choke to get the ignition fired up. As I left, the noise of my engine reverberated, waking the entire street.

Driving a car is not straightforward for me. I can only drive using hand controls, which means that I must choose a vehicle with automatic transmission. Beneath the steering wheel a lever is fitted, which I lift for acceleration or press to brake. A thick rod runs down the length of the steering column, attached at the base to the acceleration and brake pedals. A rotating ball fitted on the steering wheel and a switch to operate the indicators complete the ensemble, meaning that I steer with my left hand. With my right, I operate the push-pull lever and the indicators.

While I can drive well enough, I still have a problem: Driving as well as navigating in unfamiliar places is hellishly difficult. Each time I buy a new car, I ask for the adaptations to be fitted at or near my home, from where I can venture out without fear of getting too lost. I have to plan my route meticulously, try to memorize it, and hope for the best. I also tend to panic when I am driving on unfamiliar routes.

Thankfully, I never got lost driving into work. Taking the long road home, however, was strangely perplexing. For the first week or two, until I actually sat down with a map and worked out exactly where I was going wrong, I would take the left fork at the top of the road, which then went straight ahead, landing me in Leith docklands, stuck behind articulated lorries and heavy goods vehicles, drivers yelling. One afternoon, having left work at five-thirty, I reached home after eight o'clock.

"Did you have a nice time?" Mum asked.

"I just got back from work," I confessed. "I took a wrong turn."

Mum laughed a strange, quiet laugh. She thought I had been to see a friend for the evening. She looked oddly at me, as if understanding for the first time what a real handicap it was, not being able to navigate my way around town.

I am grateful my work colleagues did not find out. What could I have said if I had been two and a half hours late turning up for work in the morning? If I told them that I had taken a wrong turn and had no idea how to get back on track, who would have believed me? I would have been a laughing stock.

At work I recognized a familiar feeling of running to catch up. I looked about fourteen years old and dearly wished I could find some hair dye to daub distinguished gray in my hair. My clients were forever asking me if I was sure I knew what I was doing. I wasn't sure, though one thing I learned early on was to sound plausible, at all costs. For the most part I must have succeeded, as I escaped skepticism with a few shrugged shoulders.

Many of my colleagues were watching me closely as I scuttled along the corridors. They calculated how long it might be before I let them down and they could let me go. I lasted a year and five months in that job, though I don't think there was much wrong with my work. My perfectionism made sure of that. Though I was shy and entirely useless at self-promotion; though I stumbled often, tripped and fell; although I knew that I was marked for removal after my first week, when I got wind that a senior partner "thought I was unnecessary and bad for the image of the firm," it was an economic downturn that sealed my fate.

Economics gave that partner the perfect excuse he needed to delete my post. He was delighted, though he hid his glee behind a sorrowful face. I was handed my dismissal papers in a first raft of redundancies. With three months' notice, my pay, and a reference, I got off lightly. I knew they were pleased to see the back of me. I was gauche and oddly unpolitical. I often told the plain truth and could be overheard apologizing to clients, all a bit of a liability in a lawyer, as it turned out. I went home and wept for an hour or so, while my mother said there was no use for tears.

So I thought, "Where to, now?" Opening the papers in the midst of the downturn, I saw lots of jobs in distant places . . . and decided to apply for one of them, based in Orkney. Why not? There wouldn't be a stampede of applications. It was something I could try.

I had a telephone interview with the senior partner, a cheerful man who did his best to sound pleased. I was then interviewed in Edinburgh by the other chap, who reported back that he was favorably impressed. When I arrived for the final interview in Kirkwall, I descended the steps of the small airplane and was almost blown off my feet. It was raining stair rods and I was soon drenched through. With hindsight I should perhaps have taken the hint and got back on the plane. A blanket of tearful gray draped teasingly around my shoulders but I saw glimmers of sunlight in the puddles over the ground. The air smelled so sweet that I took great lungfuls of it, feeling lucky to be alive.

It was the fresh air and natural beauty of the islands that persuaded me to take my chances there. I filled my little car with my possessions and drove north to the ferry port at Scrabster. The two-hour crossing was soon behind me, and though it was raining when I arrived on Mainland Orkney, in my more optimistic moments I felt as if I had been given a fresh start.

On Main Street, Kirkwall, the sight of a strange new person—man or woman?—staggering conspicuously across wide flagstones, attracted stares. No doubt the locals knew everyone and found it odd not to be able to place me, as "yon woman who lives with Effie Sinclair's niece . . ."

Too late, I realized that I might uproot my life and move hundreds of miles, but it was not such a simple matter to leave my feelings behind. Mum sent me a postcard around that time on which she wrote, ". . . *meanwhile from you a happy letter and a sad phone call.*" In a fog, which felt like a sharp, alarming depression, I settled into life in the North with a very gentle and kind woman who made up the fire for me in the living room of her hardworking household. She cooked excellent food and filling breakfasts to fortify me against the chill, biting wind, and rain. Taking up a new position in January was brave. I was determined to give it my best shot. I had to work hard not to cry too often or too loudly where someone might hear me.

I moved out of my comfortable room after a month into a hovel I had found in the West Mainland. If you wanted to save money to fly home every weekend, as I did, it was perfect. It was utterly doomed to fail if I was looking to settle down happily in solid comfort somewhere warm, as I should have been. I was too alone to know what I should be doing, so I buried myself in my work, which became one of my coping mechanisms, though not a very successful one.

Despite my best efforts, I left that post under a cloud, eight months after starting. Once again, on the pretext of poor performance, some excuse was found to oust me while my mentor was on holiday. "Either you jump, or you will be pushed," was how it was put to me. Though I don't think I was a hopelessly deluded lawyer whom everyone secretly knew was awful at her job, there seemed to be reason to find me undesirable. Perhaps I was making the occasional mistake or two, or I fell at someone's feet or into a client's lap. I tried to fall gracefully. Everyone makes mistakes, but to compound my sin, I was just plain embarrassing. By the time the senior partner returned, I was on my way out. A pity, but there was nothing much he or I could do.

Should I have come home? I couldn't bear to, so I stayed on and found another job working part-time at the other side of the Orkney mainland. It meant a lot of extra driving, but the quiet country roads were picturesque. I had only myself to please, so what did it matter? When I told one of my colleagues where I was going to work next, she frowned, "Are you sure that is what you want?" I should have taken the hint. I should have listened.

I went to work part-time, which I thought would suit me better. I was still living alone, still in my hovel, traveling sometimes one hundred and thirty miles a day, back and forth. That was easy, compared to what I made myself do at work. It started well, but when reality started to bite, I refused to listen as my heart spoke more and more sadly to me: *for pity's sake, give this up and go home.*

I had a room up the stairs, conveniently out of the way of the rest of the office, so that I was left to myself for hours at a time, often silently or in tears, wrestling in my eagle's nest with piles of ancient, mildewed title deeds that no one had looked at for years. I suspected that I was being handed the impossible cases in the hope that I would fail, but I refused to surrender. I worked and I got it right. Once I even sorted, with two conversations and a couple of hours' work, a case that had lain untouched for over thirty-five years under one partner's desk.

The managing partner was only rarely civil to me. I often received instructions from her at short notice and once, during my afternoon off, I was telephoned by her secretary and given instructions to go into the office to prepare a court writ the likes of which I had not seen before. No asking politely, just telling. Instead of replying "Get lost" or words to that effect, I went in after hours and sat at my desk. With a dusty volume retrieved from a high shelf, I set to work, receiving rare praise the next morning. It was testament to my perfectionism that there were so few occasions when my boss could find real fault with my work, though she was forever trying to dig out *something.*

I was bullied and harassed. More than once, the suicidal feelings that had moved at my back since secondary school erupted into a full-scale gazing-into-the-abyss crisis. I would lie on my bed during weekends with the blinds pulled down, or sit for hours in a dark fog of misery, neither eating nor sleeping. Like many youngsters, I only tolerated such deep unhappiness because I had lots of youthful energy to waste on lost causes. I was afraid to make a fuss, to admit I was doing the wrong thing. I was terrified to be without work. I dreamed of working in a café or a pub serving drinks, or in a garden center rooting in seedlings, or in a local supermarket.

Perhaps Alice thought it was acceptable to treat a member of her staff in this way, or perhaps she was doing me a favor: no one likes to work with a doormat. Eventually, she must have hoped I would react. I did, and my stock with her went up immediately.

Later I discovered that my stint of two years, nine months, and several days was something of a record. Back in Edinburgh at a seminar—in an encounter arranged by the gods—I sat next to the one man among thousands who had worked in the very post I held after him. He took me by the arm after our day's learning and we spent a very friendly hour or so exchanging reminiscences and consoling one another. He decamped with his family in the middle of the night after a year. I had set my aim for three years; I almost managed, but in the end, that small, warped ambition defeated me, though I finally did leave with a show of defiance. I felt proud of myself at last, yet I wept for days afterwards. That job cost me all my savings, all my self-respect, and every ounce of strength I had. It took me the better part of two years to recover.

Chapter Thirty-Three

During all this time I was unwillingly celibate and enduring a rather hand-to-mouth existence in shabby accommodation. I found it hard to bother eating or looking after myself properly. I spent long days playing a particularly addictive version of Patience, which I got very good at. I would sit at the table shuffling the pack while my body grew steadily colder. The fire would flicker, smoke, and die quietly and I would not have eaten a hot meal all day, but I got my game of cards out!

Along the way, I bumped into Arthur. He noticed me, and after that first connection, he found me in the street, and winked, grinning and waving in my direction. I met him at dances where he held me in his arms. He came to my front door carrying gifts, cheerful and smiling. We didn't spend many months courting, as I recall. Before long, I accepted the inevitable and we moved in together. In the North, being solitary poses extra challenges: For much of the year, a chilly wind whips across the face, catching out thin townies like me who doggedly cling to romantic notions of getting back to nature. Those who opt to live in the northern wilds understand the need for good food and warm company to fend off the endless darkness of a winter that can stretch from October to May. Dangerous wind chills make huddling together for warmth a necessity.

Though anyone looking at us would have said we were chalk and cheese, Arthur was a good man who had been down on his luck when I met him, renting a single room and feeding coins into an electric meter for light and warmth. When his money ran out, he would sleep and eat in the cabin of his sturdy fifty-foot boat, which he berthed at the pier. During summer, he used his boat to take anglers out fishing, to work at the salmon harvest, or take dive parties to visit the remains of the German fleet, which had been captured at the end of the First World War. While interned at Scapa Flow, a wide natural harbor and Royal Navy Base, the entire fleet was scuttled on the orders of the German High Command before it could be useful to the enemy. Wrecks remain scattered on the sea bed around Orkney mainland, providing an unexpected boost to the local tourism industry. Arthur was willing to set his hand to anything to make a living, especially as his work was mostly seasonal.

He also had a talent for finding value that other people overlooked. He occasionally dredged for "sea coal," the hard, industrial coal used to power steam ships at the turn of the century. When hulls were cleared out, leftover sea coal was dumped in the Flow. It burns at higher temperatures than domestic coal so with that in the hearth, we were always warm. Once, Arthur used cordite explosive retrieved from a war-time mine as a fire starter. One strand carefully set would have been enough, but he grabbed a couple of handfuls. An almighty blast in the fireplace had him in fear for his life, as all the ornaments on the mantelpiece danced and the dog fled to safety behind the sofa.

What struck me most about Arthur was his optimism. His quiet sense of purpose was impressive. He worked incredibly hard, long hours, setting his wits and strength to the next money-spinning project. I would learn from him, eventually, that no matter how hard life is, there is always reason to hope for better things.

He was rather surprised that I took up with him and so was I. But something in his expression caught at me and held on. I saw in his eyes a deep appreciation for what I could do. He was unprejudiced. Nor was he swayed by the way I looked, talked, or moved. He was the first man I lived with, and though our love life was sporadic and subdued, somehow that didn't seem to matter much. Whatever way we arranged it, we had enough mutual affection and regard to be getting on with, and lived companionably together for two years. I helped him get back on his feet, and he helped me to grow up.

However, in the community where we lived, our togetherness was the subject of curious questions and puzzled frowns. I was a respectable solicitor, so what was I doing, living with a rough grafter who had a reputation for sailing close to the wind? More folk than I realized at the time were judging us by appearances. A concerned, motherly colleague took me aside to ask, just to check that being with him was what I really wanted. Was I sure? Yes, I was sure enough. They saw his rough exterior. I saw his strength of character, optimism, and intelligence.

Meanwhile, I was earning barely what I needed to make my work worthwhile. I put in many more hours than I sought pay for, and my difficulties with the demands of the office escalated. I was grateful I had someone else to think about, though even with Arthur's companionship and optimism I was not an easy woman to live with. He did his best to cheer me up, and his care and affection for me showed in touching and beautiful gestures: our Christmas trees he so lovingly hung with a web of twinkling lights and tinsel; the waistcoat he found for me that fitted and suited me to perfection and kept for many years; the two large cast-iron bathtubs that he set, one to each side of our front door and filled with earth and a riot of bright flowers. But by now, chronic depression was my intimate friend, a slobbering black dog hanging over my shoulders, remorselessly demanding my attention, though I had none to spare for walkies.

My doctor was getting fed up with me. There was only so much he could do for a woman who refused to make her own peace of mind a priority. I had my first real breakthrough when a sympathetic psychiatric nurse suggested that I might like to try my hand at art therapy. I started desperately pouring out and stirring vast pools of bright paint onto sloping sheets of paper. Only then did I start to notice just how confined I had allowed my life to become. After a weekly hour of colorful freedom, I would crawl back into my Mini and gradually fall back to earth, shrinking my ambitions to their usual gray shade and small size.

How sorry I feel for inflicting hard, cold mountains of pain on myself, all because I felt less than perfect. In being cruel to myself and by allowing others to be cruel to me, of course I became a cruel woman: sarcastic, critical, resentful, sharp, full of judgments, and unforgiving. I was all these things, and I hurt myself most of all on my jagged edges. I did this to myself. I took the blame. Unable to defend myself against even the most outrageous suggestions, unable to know what to say, when or how to say it, I was squeezed by my own self-hatred and the relentless expectations of others into a shape I no longer recognized.

Anyone who is constantly hedged with restrictions or crushing compromise will either learn passivity or rebellion. All children will gain their independence eventually and can, if they are able, walk away and start afresh. For those of us less able to take ourselves away, a different outcome is more common: frustration and anger turn inwards, where they slowly destroy.

To leave aside any pattern of failure requires an act of faith or a hand up from someone who is not tied to the painful past. Though I did not know where that help would come from, there was something within me that refused to surrender. Doing art therapy gave me a glimpse of what is possible when we allow ourselves to express our feelings and dream.

Chapter Thirty-Four

It is painful to see all the mistakes of my past parading before me. It is sad to admit that for more than half of my life, I found my sole purpose in trying to please other people. I thought that if I could please them, I would be loved. Why did I think that would work? Time and again, I found myself in barren, painful, and worrying circumstances because I discounted the worth of my own choices so completely that my life dwindled to nothing.

The other members of my family were getting on with their lives: Elouise had put down roots in Wales; Simon had been summoned years earlier to complete his Belgian national service, after which he decided to stay on and work in Brussels; Martha was in a happy long-term relationship and working as a doctor in posts all over Scotland. Yes, she is a doctor. Perhaps she was persuaded by my mother that, with her good grades, anything else would be a waste of time. Martha is a nurturing soul, whose patients love her.

In contrast, I resolutely set aside my preferences for any obvious, happy solutions, as if I was trying to prove I could manage the impossible, and no one dared to try and stop me. I was so obstinate and where did it get me? For many years I was paid dirt-poor wages simply because I didn't have the courage to ask for what I earned. It's funny, really, people could barely hide their resentment, since everyone "knows" that lawyers are lazy, opinionated, and paid far too much for doing nothing. One man, with whom I was enjoying an interesting chat about ecology, the environment, and sustainable fishing, turned his back on me when I let it slip that I was a solicitor.

"Soliciting" is demanding and difficult. I am proud that I managed to work at it for ten years. Twelve-hour days are fairly routine and it helps if you can do three things at once without taking proper refreshment, meals, or rest. Unfortunately, at that time, part-time posts were rather thin on the ground and it was a challenge to find suitable openings. Those that were suitable were obviously less lucrative, while, as I was discovering, my contracted hours had a habit of stretching uncomfortably. If I was to have any hope of not becoming exhausted, part-time posts became my only option. I knew I would only be able to sustain working part-time if I resolutely refused to do extra hours and asked for what I was due in wages. I failed dismally on both counts, routinely putting in far more hours than I was paid for, which defeated the point. On part-time wages, working cost me money I didn't have.

Frightened and believing that I was destined to live a life in which choices were a rare luxury, I flitted uncomfortably in and out of work, like a moth that moves too close to the light only to panic and flee as its wings singe in the heat. I did not know what I would rather do, and I never made space or time to ponder this for myself. It was only when I was forced, by illness, depression, or unhappiness to confront my failures that a short breathing space would appear. Even then, I failed to make the best of these respites and would snatch only a small, panicked breath before diving headlong into the next trial and error.

Chapter Thirty-Five

I had my first encounter with complementary medicine during my time in Orkney. At work I noticed that my back and neck had started to seize up, to such an extent that over a period of months I found I could no longer bend down. Getting dressed was difficult and putting on socks and shoes took me several breathless minutes. Because the twinges, aches, and pains came and settled over me gradually, I assumed that such decrepitude was only part of getting older, though I was not yet thirty. When I consulted a doctor, I was given painkillers and told that was all he could do for me. I wasn't sure, so I kept the doses low and hoped for the best.

I happened to fly home for the weekend and in the course of a morning with Mum, she couldn't help noticing how hard I was working to put on my shoes. She looked on as I sweated and swore, and then commented, "It's not normal, you know, not to be able to tie your shoelaces! You need the help of Dr. Bannerman." She telephoned his practice and was granted an immediate appointment, if I could get myself dressed and there within the hour. I was impressed and tearfully grateful.

Dr. Bannerman gave me a hard massage, manipulation, and gentle traction. At the end of our session, he stressed that I would feel very tired, as my back had been stretched and put into a better alignment, so all the shivering nerve endings in my body would need time to adjust. I felt heavenly, euphoric. I was on a high. The accumulated stiffness and pain of years was dissolved with massage lasting half an hour.

The pain during the week that followed was divine, because it was the right sort of pain: corrective and healing. It was a revelation to me that there can be such a thing as healthy pain. This understanding has helped me to identify which pain is a nuisance and which pain is healing, so that I can deal with dangerous twinges early, while trusting myself to go through "good" pain rather than trying to avoid it.

After a week of resting at home, I returned for another half-hour appointment of minor adjustments; and that was that, more or less. I was sorted and could walk, sit, bend, and raise myself up easily. I was about an inch taller. I could hardly believe it. Relief washed over me. I wanted to fall flat on my face at the feet of this miracle worker and become his groupie, but Dr. Bannerman seemed to hardly notice that what he did was miraculous to me.

I was advised to get occasional checkups to avoid a similar backlog in future. You bet! I didn't need to be told twice, and left clutching his note of useful names and addresses like a talisman.

Noticing how it felt to sit at my workstation after a session of massage, I became aware that work stress had a habit of sitting on my neck and shoulders, before slipping down my back. I began to notice how tension affected my body, and to choose to sit, work, and breathe differently, so that I caught warning aches early and made changes quickly. The health benefits of my new awareness have been incalculable.

As I began to understand that stressful conditions translated into back pain, I woke up to the knowledge that, for health reasons I had not before considered, working in an office in difficult conditions was a mixed blessing. Was it worth working so hard to keep a job, if the end result was endless pain and inability to function? Back pain is still regarded as difficult to treat successfully. What could I do? These questions, and many others, needed answers.

Chapter Thirty-Six

August was warm and bright when, once again, I returned home heaving my single suitcase and a sigh of relief. This time I knew I was home for good. In my right hand I carried all my worldly possessions, including four clay bowls that Martha had crafted for me. In my rush to leave, at the last moment I also remembered to pack a couple of books. The rest was clothes, mostly old, dusty, and dilapidated. At the age of thirty-three, I didn't have much to show for my life. Standing outside the front door of my mother's flat, memories of my hasty flight from the North made my eyes mist over.

I had spent the previous three weeks crying desperately, leaning my back against dry stone walls in the open air. Out there I hoped no one would hear my racking sobs except perhaps nesting curlews and agitated lapwings. As I left that life behind, I stood to the rear of the ferry, which smelled so sweetly of salt and oil, waving goodbye to Arthur who was not right for me, and his dog. They watched, their faces tilted sadly into the sunshine, as anguish streamed down my cheeks unchecked.

Arthur loved me and I loved him, but by now I was jammed into a corner: I knew I was going nowhere, downhill fast, and I had to look to my future. Though the severance from him felt like a bleeding arm, we both knew that I had to leave Orkney and get a life. Since walking out of my job, I had occupied myself by, among other things, helping to run Arthur's business affairs. I was frustrated and driving him up the wall. I was broke and lonely. I could no longer ignore the truth that I needed more than football, fish, and dirty jokes in my life. I needed music, conversation, and a gentleness that had got lost in our business-like relationship. I was sad to be leaving, but had to make other plans.

Beneath the sorrow of that loss lurked another treacherous love affair that turned my stomach and sent my brain spinning madly. Julian, an otherworldly man who used several different names, was everything that Arthur was not, hence the attraction: tall, elegant, well-spoken, amusing, with impeccable taste and a beautiful laugh. Our eyes first met and understood, twinkling in shared humor across a wide room. The other people around us carried on talking and we ignored them. I barely noticed his thin frame wrapped in elegant cashmere with fraying sleeves. He walked carefully. Lightly, he invited me to his house, and fool that I was, I took myself there in the car that Arthur had bought for me and brought up from "sooth."

We hugged, laughed, kissed, and held hands. Our palms met and matched. I felt understood. Before any relationship could be established, Julian lobbed uncomfortable revelations about his life and the state of his marriage into our polite conversation. I identified with his pain, so I let him talk, trying not to look too shocked and thinking what a sheltered life I had led. Murders, beatings, and suicide all found a place in his story, casually mentioned between sips of tea and the offers of biscuits, homemade, of course. I did not think I could leave him alone with his torments. Before long, I loved his voice and enjoyed my role as listener. We had relaxed conversations in his glass room at the back of the house. Now I noticed he was very ill and tiptoeing everywhere.

I bought bags of food for him and drove the slow miles to his house, knowing he would be watching my car from his front yard. I wept for the thinness eating away at him. There was nothing I could do to help, but I tried, anyway. From my meager pocket I later paid for visits to his masseur, who looked down his nose at me while I waited for the appointments to finish. Julian laughed with him.

Gradually, I saw revealed beneath the elegance and a beautifully ordered household, a fretful voice full of opinions. Opinions delivered in a gentle, cultured voice added gravitas. His light repeating that I could not stay, that there were other things to do, other people to see, his words told me that I was in the way. With a shock, I heard his opinion, so quietly offered, that I was "borderline manic." I spun this way and that in a disbelieving panic, before fleeing, knowing that his talents, his house, had seduced me. Arthur was watching in the van outside, while my world collapsed. He was devastated too, though I did not see that at the time. I felt only loss, emptiness, and the agony of another choice gone wrong.

Quietly, I took myself away and blessed the house I left behind, the gentle click of the door latching me out. I could not return to Arthur, so I spent the weekend at my favorite guesthouse where I had first found such a warm welcome, weeping, afraid that my mind was imploding, before I found refuge house-sitting for a friend who was going on holiday for two weeks. Karen has never known that her offer to house me gave me the space I needed to gather up some vestiges of dignity from the shards of my failures. What is the attraction in dangerous liaisons? Perhaps that for a while they make us feel vivid, alive.

Julian said he loved me—he may have, I'm still not sure. I think he could not resist playing damaging games with my head because he was dying a lingering, painful death. Dancing with cancer, he became careless of the hurt he caused in passing. But the contrast his life offered with what had gone before, that was Julian's gift to me, after all.

So I was home again. I thought I had failed and that my years and months away "by myself" were bound to show up as a loss on my balance sheet, but, with hindsight, I am not so sure. I certainly learned a lot more about how painful life is when we make all the wrong choices for all the worst reasons. Girls, if you want to know where to get good advice, go to the woman who loves you. Find one who treats you gently. Find a gentle woman and just listen.

My sister Martha was very gentle with me and I didn't listen to her. She didn't ask me directly, though with every gesture and sign she spoke kindly, saying, "What are you doing here, in this dump? Why do you stay here, by yourself? Why not just come home?" Her brow crinkled in a puzzled frown. When she visited me, she worked to make my current hovel homely, by baking bread, serving delicious meals, and doing the dishes, so that I could relax and try to see the world through eyes refreshed by real love. We went for long drives in the car under windy skies to distant cliff tops, and peered over ledges at birds' nests and swooping fulmars playing their outstretched, rippling wings over updrafts at the edge of giddy overhangs.

The air in Orkney is achingly sweet and clear and I love the place— it was just my life that was a mess. I realized after so many years alone that I could not fix anything there, by myself.

My life was back at a beginning, and this time I had to get it right. By trying to live according to what I believed was expected of me, I was failing because too many of those expectations were contradictory and impossible. Perhaps it was time to stop trying so hard. Perhaps if I just let go for a while, life would find a way to pick me up and carry me along on a gentler tide.

Chapter Thirty-Seven

A few days after I returned home, I decided that I was having "at least a year off from all men." I made this decision as I got off the bus, on my way to help out at a legal advice clinic run by the Citizen's Advice services. With that bright resolution to strengthen me, I immediately felt lighter, happier, freed from old bonds of sorrow. For once, I decided I could simply please myself. What a feeling! As I wandered up the steps of the office, in the late sunshine, the optimism that had deserted me for years flared up and I felt excitement.

I pushed on through the main door into the front office, and there, sitting, eating a packet of chips and slurping on an illicit carton of Ribena, was Eddie. I knew we were not supposed to eat or drink in the front office. I recognized a fellow rebel. When his eyes met mine, I was feeling as light as a feather. I fell in love with him, standing in the doorway, just like that. My resolution to take time off from men lasted all of thirty seconds.

When Eddie offered me a lift home after our stint, I offered the usual abrupt, "No, thank you," but for the entire slow journey home on the bus, my heart was remembering how wonderfully he smiled—a real smile.

I gave up the volunteering lark after a couple of months. It was too complex for an arrogant newcomer such as me. Many "hard cases" came into this office, since other "softer" options had already been exhausted. By now I had found a part-time job, which—here we go again!—was starting to consume more of my time. Two weeks after I had started my new job, that same gentleman with the wide smile sought out my number and phoned me at work. He said, "You stopped coming!" and asked me to go on holiday with him, to Orkney from where I had just escaped. He had no way of knowing I was still traumatized, that a sentimental attachment to these beautiful islands was the very last thing on my mind. So I had to say "No, thank you," and after two rejections, I was sure I wouldn't see Eddie again.

I tried not to think about him. I made excuses to myself: I really did not want any more painful, emotional entanglements for the time being. I was going through a busy time, filled with the everyday details of finding a new life, settling into my new job, finding somewhere to live. I was back staying at home with Mum, though we both knew this arrangement could only be temporary. After I moved to my present home, I worked out that I had flitted twelve times in ten years. Unsurprisingly, there was usually something better for me to do than dwell on Eddie's wonderful smile, his soothing voice, and gentle kindness.

I knew we had many things in common: We had both attended fee-paying schools in Edinburgh (which neither of us enjoyed); he had lived all his life in the city and had a degree in law from Edinburgh University. He had a quiet, self-effacing intelligence and we both enjoyed verbal sparring, though he taught me the importance of gentleness, of not getting carried away and being unkind, just to make a point.

He even helped me without realizing: to find a flat I thought of checking where he lived and then looked for something in the same area. I didn't plan to be near him, necessarily. I just knew that the area he had chosen would probably suit me, too. It did. I ended up living around the corner from him in a two-room apartment that my parents paid for.

God, it seems, had plans for us. When we first met, Eddie spilled his Ribena all over the desk where we were sitting, threatening papers and files, so that I quickly whipped out my large white handkerchief to mop up the liquid. I did not want this nice young man to get a telling off. Later, I absentmindedly put the handkerchief in a wash with my white work shirts, which came out a pretty light pink, so that for six weeks, while the color faded, I thought of him every time I put one on and in any daydream moments while I was working. As I hung my laundry outside, I could just see the rear of Eddie's flat. It was not possible for me to forget him, even if I had wanted to.

For the remainder of that year and throughout the next, as we met up, at first on gentle dates and evenings out, we gradually got to know each other. It was fun to hang out the windows and wave, or sit on the sofa talking and giggling. I enjoyed greeting Eddie at the door and acting the wife. A friend of his, who lived across my street, told him that whenever he saw me pulling down the blinds and switching on the lights, he knew Eddie was expected. The rest of the time, I watched the night sky and waited for the blue nights to close in, quite happy to sit with darkening shadows.

I have to thank my failed heating for the fact that we finally got together. That second winter felt particularly icy and my apartment had no radiators. I suppose successive owners had considered the small rooms in the apartment and decided that any investment in central heating was hardly worthwhile; but, facing north west, and built in red sandstone, my home had little natural light and felt chilly even during the summer months. That January, it was so freezing that even the mice left, casting their eyes sadly in my direction as they disappeared in search of somewhere warmer to sleep. I wore my coat, hat, and gloves indoors, as did Eddie when he ventured over. Then, when I needed its miserable ration of warmth most, the "real flame effect" gas fire I had inherited flunked out on an expensive part that would take weeks to order and install.

My living room had kitchen units at one end, so I reasoned that the whole room could be kept warm with the help of the oven. I lit the gas, but on that chilly afternoon, no flame leapt up to warm me, so I was forced to call out the gas men, who came round and immediately condemned my cooker, slapping red stickers all over the front, "Condemned appliance: do not use!"

"But how am I to cook? How do I stay warm?" I asked, shivering.

"Not our problem, pal!" they answered as they left, grinning and running down the stairs.

I had been staying at Eddie's place more often, so it didn't take much to persuade me to abandon my humble lodgings and move into his warm flat and his warm life. As I crawled like a frozen stick into his warm bed, he wrapped his cozy arms around me and I knew I was where I belonged.

Chapter Thirty-Eight

When Eddie first asked me to marry him, he actually got down on one knee. In the restaurant where he seemed to hold a season ticket, the staff watched and smirked with gentle pleasure as, with his tie all askew, he knelt with a wobble. "You know what I'm going to ask?" he croaked self-consciously. "Yes," I answered quietly, wondering whether a girl being proposed to was supposed feel euphoric, or what? He looked foolish and endearing, and I knew that beneath my numbness, my hurt, and the many bruises I carried, there rested a genuine calling out to his love. I immediately said "yes" again to his question, though, deep down, a part of me still wondered who he was talking to. He repeated his proposal several times with no kneeling, so sure was he that I would change my mind. I have never had any serious doubts.

I sold my two elegant, cold rooms with indecent haste, so that Eddie and I could make a new warmer, brighter home together and marry. I am deeply grateful to my parents for providing the financial security for us to begin a new life, and for trusting me to choose well. I know that without their material provision for me, any "normal life" I might have reached for would have been as remote as the moon.

It was a time of transition for us all. Around that time, my father retired and returned to live in Belgium. My mother sold her flat in Edinburgh and moved to France, where she lives happily. At the same time, Martha went with her husband to Australia where he had arranged to do a work swap for a year, leaving me once again without members of my family nearby. After urging me to come home, my family was now moving away in opposite directions. If I didn't know them better, I might have been quite upset. Perhaps this was their way of saying I could manage now that I had a strong, kind lover in my life.

Eddie didn't know the half of it. Though I had a job, I was scarcely earning enough to do anything so frivolous as buy a cup of tea in a café or go out for a night on the town. Heaven knows how I would have coped if I had needed to pay rent or a mortgage, like other people do. I continually made excuses for my groveling, my poverty, and the endless, shabby compromises I put up with. I reasoned that I was so grateful to be working: *"For a bully?"* my heart asked. I fobbed off these whispered warnings. I refused to accept that this employment, which I started with such good intentions, was becoming unhappy because, though I was in my early thirties, I was still frightened to say "no" and mean it. I wasn't exactly a coward, but I had a permanent feeling of being less than worthy and groveling, especially to anyone who wielded authority over me. I hated to admit I was wrong, so I stuck where I was, at a loss.

At one stage, I calculated that I was earning seventy pounds for a fifty-hour week. I totted up my taxable income for the years previous and present, and it came to less than the annual tax-free allowance. Was I mad? Possibly. When I went looking for extra income in the form of top-up benefits, the chap at the other end of the phone line asked, "So, let me get this straight, you are working a fifty-hour week? For seventy pounds, you reckon . . . ?" When I agreed, he put the phone down on me. Either he didn't believe me, or he was trying to tell me that if I was prepared to do that, there was nothing he could do to help me. I had to sort myself out first. How right he was, though I could add that when your options are limited and you are judged by appearances, you will put up with all manner of indignities just to make ends meet, just to try and fit in.

In my precious spare time, I was writing poetry on scraps of paper while I did an honest job and tried to vary my routine now and then. Nothing drastic, just leaving promptly at five of an evening, not working on weekends, and not trying to do a whole week's work between three and five on a Friday afternoon while clients handed down instructions from the golf course and the boss was away at yet another stag weekend.

Eddie and I were in no hurry to tie the knot. We enjoyed being together peacefully; laughing, dining out, going to the cinema, meeting his family and getting to know them. I loved Eddie's mum the first time I saw her: Izzy stood up when I first came into her kitchen, very formal and worried for her younger son. Perhaps falling in love is catching, I thought, as I saw her bright eyes and honest face. She had a wonderful laugh, a willing chortle. She taught her son well: he is honest, kind, loyal, and loving, just the man for me.

Though Izzy was very pleased, we soon discovered that our engagement was not greeted with universal rejoicing. My mother thought I would do better living the single life, keeping things simple and staying in touch with my friends. How little she knew me. She was blissfully ignorant that I had spent most of my years as a single adult, gripped by fear and a harrowing depression made so much worse by being alone. Fear spirals out of control when we have no one with whom to laugh.

With Eddie to strengthen me, now I could say, let others run in circles of confusion, divided and fretting over our decision to marry. What difference would that make to me? Conflicting pieces of advice flew around my head like strange, dark moths, dusty shadows trying to blot out the light I had found. In the storm of opinions, I learned to listen politely to every word, to say a quiet "thank you," and then choose the bits that felt good.

Marrying Eddie is the best thing I ever did. Any time I have any doubts, I just have to look at him to know that he loves me and I love him and that everything is fine. Our life together is wonderful. Anyone who harbored uncertainties has by now been totally won over by Eddie's constancy, my mother included. I know that surrendering to happiness with him saved my life. Anyway, what girl in her right mind would turn aside from true love?

Everyone in my family was at our wedding, which was organized for the year end so that there would be no clash of summer timetables. My father had only met Eddie the day before we got married, yet with tact and good humor he blessed us completely and gave me away with graceful charm. I was so proud of him. As we moved nearer to each other so carefully, we rediscovered our gentle affection for one another. My mother dressed up to the nines for the big day and was quiet and reflective until later that night, once the jazz got into its swing. Then my mother smiled, sang, and danced. The omens were looking good!

I did not want or need a white wedding, so Eddie wore his best kilt outfit, and I chose a dark, well-cut suit in gray wool. A strange choice, perhaps, but where was I going to keep a wedding dress? For once, I had a genuine reason to buy a really good outfit, and I took the chance to purchase something handsome and useful. No doubt, there were jokes about who was wearing the trousers in our marriage, but I only wanted to dance freely to the jazz band! All my friends came to our party, from the south, the north, and from Orkney. The love in the room that day was overflowing and genuine—the best gift we could have had to start our lives together.

My parents were brave to bless me so cheerfully since they knew I could hardly be trusted to act in my best interests. Despite their reservations, even they could see that Eddie had a calming, gentle, and firm way that I responded to gratefully. We had a truly happy party, knowing that for once I was being selfish and doing the right thing: marrying the love of my life.

Chapter Thirty-Nine

It can be no coincidence that, as I skidded into my later thirties, with my physical vigor on the wane and with a husband like Eddie to nudge me towards a gentler perspective, my painful pursuit of the law finally began to lose its appeal, though it took me a year or two longer to admit that I was never going to catch the dream—I don't mind if you call me slow on the uptake! It was always going to be a painful admission: There go twenty years of my life, right down the pan. That loss cut into me even as the binds of my pursuit were loosening. I was grieving for a career in which I had spent so much of my life and which I was now desperate to escape.

Having left the boss who liked to start his weekends early, I had found another job. All too quickly, I found myself tired, then exhausted, then despairing, and still I worked. Each day as I ventured to town, parked the car, and reached my seat in the basement, I would fantasize about breaking out, leaving, and never coming back. A low hum of dread settled in the pit of my stomach, but no one thing was bad enough to force my hand, so instead l lived with the fear that one day I would be found wanting, exposed.

It seems that my body was also urging me to leave, despite all the plans I harbored for self-harm and denial. One day I came home after work with such tiredness washing over me that I felt I might collapse and drown. I crawled into bed and fell into a heavy, uncomfortable sleep. By morning I had a fever and my right leg was swollen red and hot to the touch. I thought I had the flu and called the doctor, pleading for a house visit. No, I was sure I could not walk, and yes, I did think it needed to be checked soon. The duty doctor came, took one look at me, and asked, "Do you have a puncture wound in your foot?" We found a tiny hole, which she examined with increasing alarm. She continued, "You have a serious infection." Opting not to send me to the hospital, instead she treated me with a double course of strong antibiotics. I spent a month with my leg up, resting, feeling like I had the flu, grateful not to be at work.

I was so blind to my own needs, that this is what it took to get me to slow down and reconsider the choices I was making. It took six more exhausting months before I finally bowed to the inevitable and quit my profession.

I don't suppose anyone can sue me for confessing that my life with the legal fraternity was not a bed of roses. Or maybe that is exactly what it was. It appeared soft and fragrant on the surface and to someone peering in from outside, I may have looked like a selfish scumbag on a gravy boat, but as soon as I tried to get comfortable—ouch! If I had been fifteen years younger perhaps disability discrimination laws might have come running to my rescue. Or maybe not. Who would want to employ an awkward pain in the neck, after all?

I was not really awkward. My plea in mitigation would have to mention that I stumbled, tripped, and fell on stones often, particularly after the first six months, when my energy began its relentless slide to the floor. That was the pattern. From seven months into any new post, my wrists routinely took a hammering on the streets, perhaps because, on top of growing fatigue, I was hurrying to work in my office outfit—black skirt, white blouse, sensible shoes with soles so thin that walking hurt my feet, though they were the best compromise I could find at the time. It was doubly hard to carry an office *persona* like "solicitor" with conviction, when I arrived for work in the morning with dirty hands, torn tights, and mud all over my shoes, having fallen a couple of times between my little car and the immaculately cleaned, wide front step of the office. My colleagues looked me over incredulously as if I had just dropped in from Mars: "Are you *sure* she is with us?"

I wasn't deliberately difficult, either. It was just that I couldn't help noticing the boss's barely contained impatience and dislike whenever I was twenty minutes late for work in the morning. In my last "part-time job" I was supposed to start at nine-thirty and finish at four-thirty, with half an hour for my lunch. Yet, the demands of the job had to be met. Often, I had no choice but to work until after eight at night if I was to have any hope of meeting unrealistic deadlines, none of which I had the luxury of setting for myself. I may have worked many extra hours in the days before my morning lateness, but that was conveniently overlooked whenever a reprimand was brewing. My bad time-keeping went on my record, the unpaid overtime did not. The fact that others took the credit and I got all the blame was "just the way it was." Everything was irrelevant, except that I should do what I was told when I was told to, no matter how unreasonable or downright impossible any instructions handed to me from on high might be.

If my energy was on the wane and I was finding it hard, I had better not ask for permission to have my hours rearranged. When I did ask—please could I reorganize my time in the office so that I might take a day off during the week to rest?—twice the partners were consulted and the reply came back, "We hope you are not telling us your work is substandard?" I got a dressing-down just for asking. Howzat for a cleft stick? I shrugged and knew then that my departure was inevitable. I waited, like a rubber band pulled too tight, that knows it must snap.

One morning, I found myself struggling—as usual. In this office the main weapon of choice was the email system, where my line manager daily planted bombs such as, "Can we have a chat when you come in, please?" These meetings took place somewhere comfortless like the coffee kitchen, where there were no seats. There was no time for rest or understanding; there was only more disapproval or another sharp rebuke, more disappointment. I knew that if I had to rise tomorrow morning, to come in to any more of this, I would die. I simply could not stay parked at my desk in the basement another minute.

At times like these, my stubbornness occasionally works in my favor to rescue me, so that I walk out rather than endure any more pain. Though that meant facing an uncertain future, the alternatives were not attractive: Who wants to jump out of a window? I clung to my hope that there must surely be other ordinary, affectionate people out in the real world, some of whom I might get to know, if I weren't stuck in a backstreet basement doing filing.

Abandoning everything, I whispered the first thing I could think of that would not raise eyebrows. I was going for a short walk round the block to clear my head. Instead, in a turmoil of distress, I pulled myself along to the main reception desk and asked to see the human resources manager. In her office, away from my tormentor, I sank onto a sofa and sobbed, shards of anger and distress pelting all over the place. I swore I could never go back or endure any more bullying, misunderstandings, or loneliness. At the time I took huge comfort in knowing that my unhappiness was only partly to do with me: I was only the latest in a line of employees. I had watched the line growing shorter, inching towards me, while I sat like a rabbit frozen in the headlights. Now, I had done my last stint as the hopeless office hopper. I begged to be allowed to go home, so my handbag was retrieved for me by a kindly woman and I left, crying.

For the first thirty-something years of my life, I did an awful lot of crying. What a waste of time that was. Where my career was concerned, I could no longer ignore the truth, which was by now jumping up and down, screaming: for pity's sake listen to me! For twenty years I had careered in the wrong direction. I had to go back, all the way to square one—immediately. I must not pass go or collect £200. I must not ask "What if?" and fill my precious future with regrets for my wasted past. Twenty years after I set off down the Wrong Path, I finally admitted my biggest mistake and turned aside, looking for another way.

I take great consolation in the realization that I didn't wait until I was past child-bearing age to wake up to reality, though as things turned out, it was a damn close call. My mother still says that if I get hard up, all I have to do is go back to the office as a temp or a freelancer. Occasionally, I meet someone who seems to believe that I was a fool to leave behind the lure of riches untold. Riches, did I say? Yes, perhaps. If I had been the right height, the right sex, the right shape . . . not the groveling, staggering maverick I turned into. If you were like me, it was going to be thankless.

What might I have done with my life, if my inheritance had been different; if I had been me, but not born into a clumsy body? With the courage that a strong frame might have offered, perhaps it would have been easier to follow a path I chose. I might have been a backing vocalist, a dancer, an artist working with huge canvasses, splashing bright splotches of cerise, teal, and gold paint. I might have been the mother of lots of children, not simply the solo miracle that is my gift from God. If I'd had more courage, I could have studied where my talents led me: art, philosophy, languages, history, environmental studies. I might have worked my way across the world. Had I not been so frightened of the jumps into the unknown—I might have danced with them!

But somewhere within me there has always rested a core of strength; and imperceptibly, rays of sunlight were beginning to penetrate my sense of gloomy hopelessness. I began to notice that, as I made changes with my own happiness as a guiding light, by slow inches my life was moving in stronger currents of my own choosing which *felt good*. I was rediscovering how good it felt, to feel good. The thawing in my heart was gathering strength. Very soon, everything was going to change again, because in the first few weeks after I left lawyering for good, I got another career. I became pregnant.

Chapter Forty

With hindsight, I know that Eddie and I were fantastically lucky. The first time we seriously contemplated parenthood, life looked down at us and smiled kindly. It did help knowing that, for once in my life, I didn't care if I got pregnant. What a feeling! I finally found the courage to do something inspired. Instead of trying to prove myself to strangers who would never be convinced, I was given the chance to be happy with Eddie and I chose that. Having our daughter is the other best thing we have ever done. Even so, I don't think I would ever suggest it was plain sailing . . .

Right in line with my non-existent expectations for happiness, I assumed and often repeated, "I will not get married." Once I got married, I automatically changed my record to "I will never have kids." Elouise and Martha both gave birth to children at this time, born only three weeks apart. I looked on with pleasure at their joy, while resolutely refusing to consider that I might one day hold my own child in my arms. While Martha kept dropping hints, "So, Fran, you don't think you will have kids, eh?" and winked at me as if she knew better, I resolutely contradicted her. She once told me that she had dreamed of me with a golden-haired girl. Yet I denied her. Why was I so willing to cast myself in the role of "Fran-Never-Have"? Simply, that is what I had come to expect—nothing.

My feelings concerning my sisters' babies were muted. I was proud, pleased, and happy for them, and to be an auntie, but by not getting too involved, I hoped to dull a sense of loss, which is bound to make itself felt when everyone else has something you desire but which you believe you cannot have. There had been far too many occasions in the past—thousands!—when I had hoped for something which did not materialize, for me to feel especially unhinged by the prospect of childlessness: I was only adding another "can't" to the pile I had accumulated and rarely stopped to ponder how that made me feel.

When I hold myself apart from others rather than risk the feelings of loss and impotent anger, which surface when I repeatedly try and fail, a gray, sludgy numbness comes and sits around me. What I most desire is fizzing excitement and exuberance which feels like bright colors. Thankfully, not everyone has held such low ambitions for me as I did. There have usually been one or two brave souls prepared to remind me what I am capable of and who trust me to make adventurous choices; who will take beautiful risks with me. They planted seeds on my behalf, which have grown very slowly and taken root.

When I first suggested to Eddie that I didn't think we would have children, I was simply repeating my old record. Of course he had not heard it before, so he sat in shock, holding my hand. His face suddenly became deeply lined and his cheeks sagged as though he was going to cry. He looked very old. I will never forget that expression, which spoke so eloquently of his desire for children, though with his unfailing gentleness he only answered, "I will go along with whatever you decide." With typical selflessness, his main concern has always been for me and for my health.

Strange to say, but along with every other personal choice I have made, once we were married, the question whether we would have children soon became an item of public property, everyone holding a strong view and few refraining from expressing it. Do able-bodied persons have to put up with such public discussions of their intimate choices? Are their private lives considered public? Are their personal competencies so often questioned? Somehow, I doubt it, whereas I felt our families watching our footsteps closely. Izzy fixed her son with her beady eye and said to him in a quiet moment, "You be careful with Fran!" which meant that he was to make very sure I did not get pregnant. After Eddie told me about this, I felt violated, appalled that his mother had spoken to him like this, in a way that she hoped I would not discover, as if it was none of my business.

Because of Eddie's assumption that I could have a child, and that it was acceptable and normal to try, I began to understand that I also had the right to take risks, to experiment and make mistakes. I have the right to get it wrong, the same as everyone else, without being criticized and rebuked for steeling my nerves to try. What kind of life would a cautious residue of expectation have left for me, otherwise? Not much of one. I can see me sitting alone, in a cold singleton flat, trying desperately to care what I eat today, and wondering who I could telephone.

Unless we are brave and take small risks, there is no way to escape the limited expectations of others. Martha's hints lit a long fuse, Eddie's gentleness gave me courage, while Izzy reckoned without my defiance. Thanks to her, I immediately began to think seriously about having children. Perhaps it was part of God's plan to place me among elders with sharp opinions so that I would feel driven to prove them wrong. When someone says, "You can't do that!" I automatically think, "Oh, yes I can!" and I go all out to prove it. I feel driven to push past a helplessness that threatens to swamp me and which so many others appear to believe is my only inheritance.

Martha was on the move again, returning to Australia with her husband and her young son. This time, it was her work commitments that would keep them away for almost three years. I realized that if I wanted to have a child, I had better think quickly. I knew that my age was against me. I needed something to do, and with typical contrariness, I risked getting pregnant when I could have been having a well-earned rest. Real life seems so disorganized, sometimes, yet it seems to work out in the end.

As with the many questions surrounding my marriage, once the news of my pregnancy was shared, there were endless huddled family conversations concerned with "whether Fran could manage," conversations from which I was excluded. Perhaps that is just as well, as my parents were seriously worried and sharing their worries would hardly have helped me. From the sidelines, Simon quietly lent his support, saying that I had a streak of steel in my character. Martha and Elouise shared some of these conversations and whisperings, though Elouise wisely decided against being too honest. In shocked tones she let slip, "Honestly, Mother sounds like a fascist!" and I could work out what that meant. Mum's current theory was that people "like me" should not be getting pregnant. I didn't know whether to be amused or devastated, although it may only have been a theory of hers, a personal preference prompted by worry for me.

I confess I set this small trap for Mum to test her reaction. When I told her I was pregnant, I asked, "D'you think I should get an abortion?" She thought for a bit, and suggested that yes, I probably should. How would I manage, otherwise? After I got off the telephone with her, my mind was quite made up. I would phone a clinic. Easy.

Then Eddie asked, "Is that what you want to do?" and I had to admit that the answer was no. I wanted to take on this challenge and see where it led me. Besides, the idea of having a termination felt wrong. I was married to a wonderful man who wanted a child. I had made the choice to have unprotected sex, after all, and as my doctor had said, "If you are old enough to have sex, you are old enough to have a baby." I knew I was facing an opportunity which would not be repeated, though I tried not to worry how on earth I would manage.

One night, I had a dream that I was up to my neck in water and drowning. But instead of running out of air, when I relaxed and let go, I was able to breathe easily underwater. Opening my eyes, I saw the tide sweeping me along in a magical underwater world of seahorses, sparkling bubbles, and colorful fish swimming past in the current. The message was clear: If I would just go with the flow, everything would work out beautifully.

Yet, though my heart understood this, in the midst of all the other practical and emotional adjustments of impending motherhood, I fretted. Looming like a ghost over everything was the feeling that my mother didn't know me well enough to really bless us. Eddie would wait patiently whenever I came off the phone with her, numbed by her recent pronouncements and he would ask, "What has your mum been saying now?" We held hands and hugged.

I never for a moment doubted that Eddie loved me and that he would be a wonderful father, but I was mired in my own fears about how I would cope, so, for the time being, my dreams and his faith would have to do for all of us. As it turned out, his faith is so great, it carried us easily.

I had a wonderful pregnancy, with not a whiff of morning sickness. Nausea, a little, though none of the endless vomiting that so nearly landed Martha in hospital. Poor Martha went through agonies of gut-wrenching sickness and the pale empty thinness that followed. She lost fifteen pounds in weight from her already lean frame. Me, I spent three months politely avoiding the cooker, nibbling dainty portions, and eating many oranges, while I tidied the apartment in readiness. I am grateful that, despite my boyish figure, my pregnancy was not obvious. I huddled away from doubters.

With no help from the antenatal services, I found out who was my allocated surgeon, unearthed his place of work, and, in his piecemeal schedule, booked myself an appointment to request a caesarean section so that I would not have the extra worry and embarrassment of wondering whether I could give birth naturally. My narrow hips, my limited flexibility would, I was sure, have made a normal delivery more difficult. There also hovered a feeling, hard to convey in words, that the midwives and hospital staff who attended me would take it for granted that I *could* stretch my legs wide, that I *could* do what I was asked. It would only be when things became too wretched that the extent of my problems would be obvious to everyone. By then, I might have to be wheeled in for an emergency section anyway. I simply do not know whether I could have given birth naturally, and no one seriously weighed up this possibility or discussed it with me. I was wary of easy assurances issued by medical professionals. Instead, it was easier to mumble that I had narrow hips and that I had no wish to inflict a birth trauma on my kid. The nurses, midwives, and doctors I visited did not pry. They understood enough and did not raise any objections, even though an elective section is rarely granted by the health authority. Perhaps, rather than publish any outright policy to this effect, they just make it difficult to arrange so that only the most determined women persist.

Instead of taking my chance to really enjoy my precious freedom to rest with my stomach peacefully, to embrace my growing child within and sing her songs, I fretted and tried to think of all the answers. Preoccupations seized me, shook me, and left me brooding and fearful. I wondered, "How on earth will I manage bringing up a baby?" When my doctor confirmed I was pregnant, she was incredibly supportive, as was the wonderful midwife, who filled the room with such palpable joy that she made me feel loved. Her many stories about her love for her own daughter were infinitely consoling and an example I could follow. I also found help elsewhere, from women and men who came to know of my pregnancy and who swore they had not the slightest doubt that I was doing the right thing. They confided in gentle whispers that of course I would manage: I would be a wonderful mum! I drew strength from such loyalty and love. We may have shared only brief conversations, quiet reassurances offered here and there, but they all added up, making a real difference to how I felt about the prospects for success.

I heard what I needed to hear—that yes, of course there are men and women who marry and who are happy and have well-adjusted children and who can still live together for decades. Yes, of course this happens all the time, it is not just the stuff of romantic fiction. And it needn't make the slightest difference that I was disabled. "Wow!" I realized, as a new truth was revealed. "You mean that I can be like you, too? It's okay to take the chance? You really think I can really manage?" From assurances I received, there grew a determination to prove that I could be a happy mother. I could join the optimists. This was what I wanted, for myself, for Eddie, and Seline. Seline—my daughter.

Chapter Forty-One

My appointment at the new hospital out of town was for seven-thirty on Friday morning, the sixth of June 2003. I was to be first in the operating theater at eight-thirty and I knew it was very important for me to be prompt. Eddie took the day off work, though we agreed that he would postpone the start of his paternity leave until after I came out of hospital. We felt odd, the two of us, with this bump resting between us as we drove away from the city against the flow of commuter traffic, knowing that our lives would be changed forever, never again just the two of us. We were inclined to move quietly, but we hurried, weaving through traffic cones and waiting impatiently at traffic lights because we were late; I, in the front passenger seat feeling absurd and Eddie at the wheel, his face set in a frown of concentration and concern, looking like a small boy.

I had been on a food fast, which meant I had eaten no food and had nothing to drink since ten o'clock the previous night, for this "major operation to my abdomen." I believed the operation would be straightforward. The only problem was, I was already hungry, though I didn't much mind. The waiting would soon be over. As we arrived and walked arm in arm along the long, quiet hallways at our new state-of-the-art facility, I felt as if I was on the moon, although we eventually found the right ward.

I hardly heard a nurse asking me, "Would you like a room by yourself?" nor did I notice her puzzled frown when I answered her without thinking, "No, thank you." I opted instead for a space in a room with four beds because I didn't want to be lonely. When Eddie and I got to the allocated bedside, I looked around the ward and saw lots of babies sleeping and having their nappies changed. What were all these women doing with babies? I still didn't feel that any of this had anything to do with me. In a daze I changed into the hospital robes, though this seemed odd: I felt perfectly well. Despite all the discussions, the videos and the silent watching of films in the dark, I felt out of it, apart. Eddie sat beside me, plied me with magazines, and we waited. And waited.

Someone who didn't tell me his name came to take my blood pressure and left. Someone nameless else came to check my history of this or that, and left. Another came to take bloods. Every hour, I heard that my op had been put back; there was another emergency in the operating theater. Okay, so I waited. At noon, I asked, could I at least have a drink? There was a long conference, and I got three thimblefuls of water in a tooth mug. Past the curtains drawn around my bed, lunch was being doled out and eaten, smells of cooking wafting. I got no food. I was feeling rather sorry for my baby and for myself too, by this time. Another youthful bloke came in after lunch and said, "We lost your bloods, and they hadn't been cross matched." So he took more blood from my arm and left. God, this was boring, I was starving, and my baby must have been wondering what was going on. Eddie was prowling, unsure when we would be called to theater and no one was saying very much. If he could wait, so could I.

At about three in the afternoon I got wind that they had just finished their last emergency section, and it would be my turn soon. No one seemed to think it mattered that I had been waiting all day having had nothing to eat since ten the previous night. I simply felt relieved.

I was wheeled into theater. You would think I would be used to this, wouldn't you? I was groggy and felt nervous and fluttery. I was given a spinal anesthetic, which took time to work. I was still asking myself why I was lying in a hospital, thinking, "There is nothing wrong with me. I feel great! I am just going to have a baby, that's all—a baby!" There were perhaps a dozen people round the table, plus Eddie in his green overalls and mask. If he hadn't been there I would have panicked. Even though I couldn't see much of his face, his eyes glinted smilingly at me as he held my hand. Thank God. I am not at all squeamish, but there is something about the smell of antiseptic and the shiny tools all sterilized and lined up ready to cut, that gets to me.

Then I heard music! As I always do, automatically I listened and heard of all things, the strains of the "William Tell Overture" on a sound system and being played rather too fast—da da *dum*, da da *dum*, da da dum dum *dum*! The man's got a head like a ping pong ball!....Wind and strings working very hard, cantering to the finish, somewhere in Switzerland. A giggle started in my stomach and wouldn't stop. Anesthetic has a relaxing effect. Grinning widely, trying not to laugh and shake all over the place, I spoke up, "Could we have some different music, please?"

"But yes of course! If you like! What do you think? Would Beethoven's Pastoral do?"

"Perfect!" said I, still laughing.

"You're the last, you see," explained the anesthetist, and indeed I could see now, that the dozen people standing around the couch were all merry and smiling. Their relief was palpable. Friday at four, and they had just finished a difficult day of complicated emergency sections, each done in a rush under immense pressure. And now, here was an elective. Easy, piece of cake. Let's get it done and get out of here: "William Tell" was the obvious choice, after all. The trouble was, I had to stop laughing. We compromised with dear ol' Beethoven. Then, I knew that everything would work out.

All I had to do was keep hold of a grain of faith. A little faith, a loving husband. I sank into the stupor and waited, while my surgeon and the anesthetists talked me through what they were doing. I didn't feel much after a second dose of anesthetic went into my spine. It takes a lot to knock me out and they double doped me. Luckily I was able to reassure them that this was normal, and after that I floated easily. I felt odd tugging and pulling. The surgeon has to work that bit harder, because all the abdominal muscles are paralyzed, put out of action by the anesthetic. After minutes that felt like an eternity, he lifted out a long, thin baby, all arms and legs. When Eddie first saw her, he grinned and blurted out, "She would make a perfect hooker!" a remark greeted with shocked silence. "Rugby! Rugby!" we hurriedly explained, so that laughter was restored, while Eddie blushed a deep shade of pink and mumbled apologies.

My baby daughter was handed over to me and I was carefully sewn up and put in the post-op room for monitoring. I felt my blood pressure sinking, exceedingly groggy, very floaty, and deeply happy. My baby was fine and while the seconds ticked past, the staff looked first worried and then reassured, as I felt myself rising up, becoming stronger, more anchored, before we were both moved gently back into the ward. Seline was nestled exactly where she should be, in the crook of my arm, as light as a feather and as silent and peaceful as an angel.

The rest of the afternoon and night, Seline snuggled peacefully in my arms, her lips fastened to my breast, her touch as light and gentle as butterfly wings. Later on during that summer evening, a nurse took her very gently from me and, in a basin placed beside my bed, washed Seline carefully in soapy warm water, then put her in a diaper and wrapped her snugly. Wash, tender wipe, dry, and wrap. I watched every tiny movement, mesmerized, still doped up with anesthetic. Seline was gently returned to me without a word. I wouldn't have known what to do, but now I was Mummy, so I watched and listened. Slowly, I would learn to do these things for my daughter, too.

I was to rest in bed after my "major operation" so Seline was brought to me, and stayed beside me on the bed during those first days of her life. The first night Seline and I were newly separate and together, I stared at her, not once closing my eyes. She slept in a peaceful cocoon, suspended in golden light. Her every tiny contour seemed blessed, minutely beautiful, crafted by a master. I whispered prayers of thanks to God, to give her health and to give me the courage to be a good mum with her, to be kind and gentle, as I could already sense she was being, with me. I swore I would protect her with my life. Nothing mattered more in that night of glimmering lights and golden beauty, than to be a good mother. I felt a strength welling in me and sustaining me with a conviction I hardly knew I could hold. She and me, we passed the night well, the two of us together entirely oblivious to the cries of other babes on the ward.

Chapter Forty-Two

The next morning, I finally got to eat. Breakfast was a tiny bowl of "Rice Krispies" with milk slopping all over the sheets and globs of rice wavering dangerously over the edge. The ration doled out was gone in three spoonfuls and I was ravenous! Breastfeeding costs extra so I begged shamelessly for more food. Perhaps that was undignified, but then, nothing about being in hospital with a first baby is dignified. While I was trying to eat as much food as possible, I quickly learnt that the cooked food we were given was often inedible: wilted bits of rolled beef and overcooked cabbage, driven up from South Wales and re-heated, anyone? It smelt awful and turned my stomach. I could feel my energies slipping, as I persisted with feeding Seline. Even I, notorious for eating large quantities of anything—I survived eight years at boarding school, after all—was unwilling to venture the fare served up and left to congeal on plates at the foot of our beds. There is no point encouraging women to breastfeed their babies while new mums go hungry on the wards. It isn't as if we can easily get up out of bed and wander to the nearest restaurant for a calorific meal.

The second night, after Eddie had visited bringing me extra supplies of food and drink, I felt lonely. My mother and father lived overseas. They were not here to see me or my baby. Martha was in Australia on her extended work contract. One of my best friends in the world had visited unexpectedly in the afternoon, breezing in like a Queen from the North, and after the euphoria she had gone again almost as quickly. As evening came, it was just me and Seline, and I felt all at sea.

The television above the bed opposite ours had been switched on and turned up to MAX all the day long. I was constantly hungry from a shortage of food, and sore from the cutting and the stitches. I told the staff on duty that Codeine made me puke, but they administered it anyway, and I threw up copious quantities of fluids and scraps of food, depleting my already thinning strength. Although it was mid-summer, the sheets felt thin. The blankets were tucked in hard and too far down the bed to offer any warmth. Someone forgot to shut the window.

After a few fretful night hours, with the lights on low, trying to feed Seline and get her to sleep while the other babies in the room cried and woke each other in rotation, I seemed to fall asleep. I jerked wide awake at two in the morning in a spinning panic. I was freezing, in urgent need of a blanket to warm myself. Seline was covered in goose bumps and crying fretfully, constantly woken out of her sleep in fits and starts by the noises of the ward. As soon as Seline, with a desperate sigh of relief, drooped in sleep, a piercing screaming from the baby in the bed next to ours tore through us like a sharp knife through air, inches away. That baby's distress and pitiful cries launched at full volume jerked Seline awake repeatedly through the night. Each fresh cry felt like a heart attack. Screaming continued until six, by which time Seline was distraught and I was utterly wretched. If any baby cried, Seline jerked awake and shuddered, turning a plea to me, her eyes brimming with sorrow. Another hour of this and I was a nervous wreck. Although I had managed to obtain a blanket and to persuade someone to please, please shut the window, Seline had not slept and was by now deeply disturbed. Every time any baby cried, she woke in a panic, so I leave you to imagine the outcome in a large, modern maternity unit. I soothed her endlessly. With tears running unrestrained down my face, I grabbed hold of a passing sleeve and begged please, please, to be moved somewhere quieter.

"Is it just your postnatal nerves my dear? Postnatal depression?" A nurse peered at me, her gentle face creased up with concern.

"No!" I whispered. "We need to get some sleep and my baby is distressed, and the television is on all the time . . ." I gabbled brokenly, beseechingly, not letting go of that sleeve for a moment, until I was swiftly moved to a better spot, away from bedlam.

Things improved a little after that. I scavenged what I could, on the lookout for what I might eat, and I carried on feeding Seline. She slept during the day, though nurses or junior doctors were forever peering at her, picking her up to take her clothes off, weigh her, measure, wash, test, and inoculate her. I began to wish that these nameless persons might at least try to co-ordinate their visits. Each time Seline was woken she grew more tired. And slept harder.

And then, in common with most other breastfed babies she started to lose weight. At four days old, there were murmurs about formula top-ups and switching over. What did I know? I wanted to ensure that she did not receive formula, but I suspect that she was given extra bottles while I occasionally slept. The old pattern of doubting came back to pester me. I was told: "This is for your own good!" and "We don't want you coming back into hospital, now, do we?" Such explanations were, I am sure, only intended to encourage me to greater efforts, but I felt pressured, as if they doubted that my boobs were up to the job.

I knew that I had to get home and that my baby and I were in danger of slipping. I was starving. If we stayed in the hospital I realized that our difficulties would only escalate and so, aware of the dilemma, I issued an ultimatum: if I didn't get more food and sleep, I would discharge myself and Seline, even against medical advice. We had already been kept in four nights. I knew that at home, with rest and food, we would both recover our strength.

I got a room to myself for one precious night. I was given extra food, salads, and meals with their vitamins intact, and things were patched up with the staff. I left the hospital on good, if not exactly cordial, terms and was invited to sign a disclaimer so that I would not be tempted to sue if it all came unstuck for me and I was looking for someone to blame. Half a dozen ward staff crowded round the bed, as if they thought I might refuse to co-operate. There was probably a party after I left.

I was so glad to get away, to go home. Walking gingerly, it felt very strange to emerge into bright June sunlight. Living under artificial lights, it is easy to forget that the rest of the world is still out there, with its soothing, healing rhythms. Eddie drove us gently, so smoothly through the traffic, as if a single jolt would fracture us all.

Chapter Forty-Three

While I was in the hospital, my new baby, like every other baby, was placed in a cot not far from my bed. One day I worked out that I would have to seek assistance because all the other mums were lifting and carrying their babies back to bed to feed them and it was clear I was expected to follow suit. I gathered my courage and haltingly explained to a passing nurse that lifting and carrying Seline was something I could not trust myself to do. I didn't want to drop my baby, I said. I had to spell it out for them, and it broke my heart quietly.

We worked out that I would have to move the cot close to the bedside, sit on the bed, lift Seline out of the cot, place her by my side, get myself comfortable, and then feed her. This was the solution I adapted throughout her babyhood, since there never was a time when I could carry my baby freely in my arms, or walk her swingingly round the house in a cozy couchette. I would have needed three arms—one spare up my sleeve—so that I had something to lean on for support. I couldn't trust my two legs to hold us up.

Father phoned me once we were home, full of love and congratulations, and asked me, what would I like? Perhaps a baby carriage for Seline? Yes, please, I said, a three-in-one would be most useful. We urgently needed to replace the clapped-out conveyance we had been given, with one with a frame narrow enough to pass through the doors of the apartment. Dad has an uncanny ability to offer the right kind of help at exactly the right time. He may go about his business quietly; and perhaps he is not here often, but he seems to know what will make the difference between success and failure. He sent me some money immediately, and the model Eddie and I chose was one of these ultra-modern contraptions with every conceivable attachment and permutation: a flexible, easy mover that, once I had learned how to take it apart and clip it together again, became indispensable to me, indoors as well as outside. I wheeled Seline around the apartment in her carriage. Later on, I used the upright seat that attached to the frame as her high chair, after I discovered that it fit neatly beneath the table where we ate, and could be washed when it got too dirty.

My life was filled with one preoccupation: how to? How to get Seline to her cot, put her down for naps or take her out for a walk in the sunshine—all these activities were subjected to "time and motion" studies designed for the woman who has mobility issues of her own. The challenges of caring for a baby at home alone meant that each and every daily activity had to be broken down into carefully manageable steps, like this:

Object: to go to the store.

Method: Mum leaves Seline on the living room floor, choosing somewhere where she will be safe for two minutes.

Mum goes to the loo, has a quick sip of water, and puts on her shoes, with baby in view. Mum ensures house keys in pocket at all times.

Mum collects shopping bag, diaper bag, and infant accessories, which she takes downstairs as quickly as possible.

Mum fetches baby car seat and, sitting down, lifts Seline into it. (Carriage cot is unsafe for lifting infant downstairs, as cot is wide, may bang on stairs, and has no strap restraints.)

Mum dismantles carriage and takes it downstairs in two trips: frame first, then cot.

Mum re-mantles carriage at foot of stairs and goes up quickly to fetch Seline.

Mum carries Seline downstairs in car seat.

As Seline gets bigger and heavier, Mum still uses car seat, but bumps down steps on bottom, or lifts car seat one step at a time downstairs.

Mum ensures carriage is near car seat.

Mum sits on bottom step and lifts Seline up into carriage cot. Car seat is left at foot of stairs for return trip.

Mum opens front door and finds something to prop it wide with. Not easy. Kind neighbor brings two pieces of wood for this use. Must remember to carry them with me, together with purse, bag, diapers, etc. Essential piece of kit for travel outdoors.

Mum manoeuvres pram over step, down, and outside.

Mum closes door.

We can now go shopping.

Mum *must not* trip or fall, though she leans on the baby carriage for support. If she trips or falls, it will catapult away from her, perhaps into oncoming traffic.

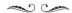

The one time I did trip and fall forward flat onto the sidewalk, an older gentleman, who happened to live nearby, may have saved Seline's life. In a manoeuvre that probably reminded him of his rugby days, he snatched the handles of her carriage as it careered towards him. I was his pal ever afterwards and we stopped for a chat each time we met. He liked to remind me of what he had done and his story made us both very happy.

While Eddie was at work Seline and I did not go out very often. Each stage in Seline's growth shifted ever so slightly the challenges of getting around with her on my own, both at home and in the world over the front door. To give one example, when Seline had a dirty diaper, the contents of which slid all up her back, I had to improvise hastily. Since this latest episode of gippy tummy had not arrived conveniently between the hours of six p.m. and eight a.m.

when I could reasonably expect that Eddie would be home, I had to find a way to carry my babe to the kitchen sink for a wash. (Using the bath was too difficult, slippery, and low down.) Was that easy? She was a long girl, heavy by then, with bowels upset during teething. I couldn't push her in a box across the floor.

I had to quickly find her car seat in the back of the airing cupboard. Although she had grown too big for it, thankfully I had kept it, since I could still use it for hoisting—just—and fetching and carrying indoors. I found a clean towel and wrapped a naked Seline up in it. Then I found a second towel to cover the car seat. I put Seline in her seat and swung her through to the kitchen one heavy step at a time. Then I lifted her hefty bod—still in the car seat—onto the kitchen counter, ran the faucets, and filled the sink with bubbles; washed her, wrapped her in the clean towel, and took her back through to the living room in the car seat, to dry and change her . . . Phew! I came to rely heavily on Eddie for help with the evening routine, and not just because by six in the evening I felt as if I have been flattened by a bus.

I had been advised at the hospital that, like all mothers who have a section, there was to be no heavy lifting for at least six weeks, and that I must take it easy, for, if I remember correctly, the following six months or so. When Eddie had to go back to work after his three weeks' paternity leave and holidays were up, I had no choice but to do what had to be done, such as lifting and carrying objects including babies, which, as is their way, rapidly grow heavier as time marches on.

Without the regular and unstinting support of some gentle women from the local church who befriended my family, we two would have been thoroughly marooned during the day. Everything felt un-nerving, raw, and I was frightened of what might happen if something went wrong and my careful preparations unraveled.

It was this uncertainty which ensured that, for the first few months of Seline's life, we spent a great deal of our time sitting indoors, feeding and sleeping together in a wide armchair that worked well for both of us. I recall two "feeding frenzies" which, if memory serves, each lasted about thirty-six hours. Was that exhausting? Totally. Was I happy? Yes. Did I sleep enough? No. I eventually decided that the only way I would stay sane was by "totting up" the hours I snatched between nightly interruptions for feeding and play, or for teething and sickness: one-and-a-half hours + two hours + seventy-five minutes = four-and-a-quarter hours. Thus, it was far easier to overlook the three or four fractures to my rest every night, as well as the early morning five o'clock starts during the light summer months. I existed in a frenzy of fatigue, but it helped when I remembered that I had nothing better to do; no pressing engagements with the outside world.

Chapter Forty-Four

Not being able to lift and carry your infant, your child, has so many practical ramifications. With each growing stage I discovered a whole new batch, which I had to work through with almost mathematical precision. Softness had to be put on hold, while I concerned myself with the one hundred and one practicalities of motherhood for which first-time mums receive no training, but which we are expected to know about, as if maternal instincts cover every eventuality: how to assemble and collapse a pram to get it on and off buses or into cars; how to pureé vegetables, and what to cook today when there has been no chance to go out to the shops; how to keep my mind active so that I didn't only think about health visitors, sore breasts, inoculations, first words, and teething troubles.

Not only were daily practicalities challenging, but with each mark of Seline's progress, fresh, sharp feelings of loss and inadequacy surfaced, catching me unawares. Shadows, which felt like mourning, sat on my shoulders. Of course I yearned to be like every other mum, to carry my daughter in my arms, to swing her up in the air as she grew older and glowed with the breathless joy of her discoveries. I wanted to run with her, jump, laugh, and skip. Instead, I hid my pain beneath the usual excuses: "I'm tired today," "I need to go and make supper," or "I would like to just sit in the sun and read my book."

All of these things I said were probably true, yet I knew I was hiding. I found it hard to admit, "I can't do that, my love, I am sorry," because when I said that, Seline looked disappointed and I had to put on my brave face, though there was a girl within me who wanted to weep. Because it was sometimes hard thinking of ways to divert her disappointment—I could hardly cheer her up by saying I would play "tig" with her later—I retreated even further into sitting and reading books.

Alarm bells were ringing. I didn't want Seline to grow up to copy me! I knew she easily might, if I could not convince her that running, dancing, spinning, and skipping are best for children. I knew that in any other circumstance, I too would be active. Movement is what I choose! The pain, fatigue, and sense of missing out often festered, making me difficult to live with.

At no time did this feel truer than during the long middle period after Seline was born, once the euphoria of her first year had worn off. Eddie was unfailingly forgiving and peaceful, but it was not enough to rely on his good nature. I knew something in me had to change, and quickly, before I became bitter and cut off. Eddie and Seline were getting the brunt of my bad temper. Sleep deprivation was fraying my mind. I could see that my little family was sinking into trouble slowly but surely, because I was exhausted, isolated, and frustrated, while I found myself in mourning for the ordinary spontaneity of mother and daughter joy. I knew that my usual coping mechanisms were due for an overhaul, though how change might come to me was unclear. There were too many difficulties and mixed-up emotions. Where could I start?

One ordinary evening, my rescue began and has been gathering pace since. I was sitting in my usual chair in Seline's room and she was still a babe, lying back along my lap, relaxed and peaceful. I suppose I must have been speaking rather crossly to her, as per usual. Then she just looked at me. Rather, she seemed to look through me, as if to say, "Mum . . . what is your problem? I am quite happy here, as you can see." She just looked through me with her piercing blue eyes and all the wisdom of ages seemed to open itself to me.

In that moment I dimly began to understand some truths that have become crucial in helping me to turn my perspectives towards a kinder, gentler way. I understood that babies and young children have no choices: they must bear with the decisions and behavior of their parents, no matter how incompetent, misguided, or harmful these may be. Seeing my own child lying quietly before me, I understood how much it meant to be responsible for Seline's nurture and care. No one else except Eddie and me could she rely on. Young infants mostly rely on their mothers. To be charged with the care of someone so small and malleable, so vulnerable, is an awesome responsibility. If I was to fulfill my promise to love and uphold her, I had to become very careful of each thing I said and did. It was totally up to me to set a good example, one which gave lots of love and wasn't afraid, but calm and softly spoken. I had to discipline myself to experiment with gentleness, step by step.

From that single look which Seline gave me, it was a jolt to realize that she could be my inspiration and my greatest teacher. My daughter's lessons were all the more powerful because she was so defenseless, yet she was unafraid of me or anything I might do.

I understood that by watching and copying my daughter's example I could discover another great lesson: when I got it wrong she was never cross with me. No matter how often I erred, she freely forgave me every time. With her, every single forgiveness was like turning over a new leaf. Here was an example I could follow.

So many mistakes we make, because we live without thinking: we build a picture with the messages and patterns we pick up as children, before we realize that simply copying the adults around us is no guarantee of success. Parents, grandparents, great grandparents. We simply repeat what they do. The only way to break those habits we would not choose, is to notice the link in the chain from mother to daughter, father to son, and decide to behave differently.

Writing allows me to see every experience in a new light and take something positive from my mistakes. In being married and choosing to have a child, for example, I can now understand the motives of those charged with my care and nurture. To understand the many frustrations and sorrows that crowded round my parents, is to recognize my debt to them, and love them more completely than ever before.

The gentleness and forgiveness that Eddie and Seline first illuminated for me as a way forward, I can gift to myself and share with others. Every day I notice I can choose. I can make amends and act with deliberate kindness, in the light of new awareness. I am learning, at last, the freedom that comes from choosing how to respond to each mistake, misunderstanding, and the seemingly random nature of life.

For me, this is the only way to stay on an even keel, because every day still carries its share of sadness and familiar longing that things might be just that little bit different: the glances of strangers who give me a wide berth in the street, warning their children sharply to stay out of my way; mothers who greet me a cheery "Hello!" and overtake, because they are in a hurry for the "school run," just as I am. At times like these, my heart fills with desire to join their careless chatter, the breezy walks past, but I don't keep up very well. I find that I have no choice except to hang behind, alone, with my old pal, a slapped on smile, for company.

Chapter Forty-Five

While Seline was still an infant, my periods became irregular and, after a bleed lasting several weeks, they dried up altogether. I was only in my early forties, though this had all the signs of early menopause. I have not had a bleed for several years now, so I take it that I am postmenopausal, at the grand age of forty-six.

That is not what I really wish to write about here, though. The reason I mention the menopause, is that passing through it has had a marked effect on what I can eat without making myself unwell, by which I mean, so sore that I cannot move or sleep. While Seline was starting to take herself places, crawling, running, and jumping with all the joy and exuberance of a two-year-old, I was finding it difficult to tolerate increasing pain in my shoulders, hands, hips, knees, and feet. A mum with a small child has to be able to walk, not crawl, and at that active age when children need to be watched closely, at the end of another long day I would be howling with the pain and sheer effort of keeping going. I was most concerned about my right foot, which takes most of my weight when I walk, so in the search for some answers and assistance I made an appointment to see a local orthopedic consultant. Perhaps, given my past experiences, I should have been more wary and kept my expectations in check.

I made an appointment with my general practitioner and went to see her, to request a referral to a specialist. I was sent a letter for a date several months later. The hospital to which I was referred is situated some miles out of town. I got there on time and sat, before being shunted to X-ray and various waiting rooms en route to my destination, the room where I would meet The Great Man. My optimism wilted. I got my first audience with the less senior doctor on duty. In the course of our ten-minute interview my hopes died as it became clear that she had not read my notes and knew almost nothing about the nature or effects of my condition. She did not ask to see me walking, nor did she listen to what I said. She implied that if I had got myself to see her, there could not be much wrong with me and that perhaps I should not waste her time. She spoke at me as if I was seven years old, but with an unfamiliar edge of hostility. To be fair, the consultant who then came in to see me had a much better bedside manner, though he blotted his copy book by suggesting that I might try wearing shoes with a slight heel.

Dazed, angry, and humiliated by the way my problems were dismissed, it dawned on me that after forty years I was bound to know more about myself than they did. I also knew that I was alone in my search for relief. I decided to use my anger to help myself.

I started reading all the books I could lay my hands on about menopause and food, what foods the older woman might avoid, and which natural foods have a reputation for combating pain. I collected lots of ideas for healthy eating, which reinforced what I already knew and strengthened my resolve. On a hunch, I cut out coffee and tea, a process which took roughly two months. It was a slow start, but every day made a difference.

Then, something made me avoid cows' milk. A memory came back to me. While I was working in town, I would go round the corner to a café during my lunch break. My meal routinely finished with a chicory drink, topped up with a generous serving of milk. As I left the café to head back up the hill to the office, I would be seized by paroxysms of coughing, which made me feel like an old man. Not a coincidence, surely . . . Cutting milk out of my diet was more challenging, because milk also includes cheese, yogurt, and butter, as well as biscuits and many baked products. After two weeks I noticed that I had stopped wheezing and scratching, and that my joints felt freer. I was on a roll so it was relatively easy to cut out refined sugar, which I had read makes pain harder to tolerate. It was an easy step from there to cutting out chocolate.

It was not just café foods that fell under suspicion, though I still find that these are the main culprits. Following a particularly painful two days as a result of eating a piece of steak, I eliminated red meat. When I made the mistake of cooking and eating sprouting potatoes, I ached all over for a day or so, which was the incentive I needed to drastically reduce my intake of potatoes as well as vegetables such as eggplant and tomatoes. A little research confirmed they belong to the Deadly Nightshade group of plants.

It makes me laugh to realize that these days my definition of living dangerously has nothing to do with alcohol, late nights, or illegal substances. I do not have much fear of death or dying but I am frightened of a lifetime of chronic pain, which helps me to remember that I had better avoid the little cubes of cheese in the house salad which taste so delicious. If I eat two portions of cheddar within a day, I will suffer for my thoughtlessness. The same can be said for most of the foods I have largely eliminated so that I cautiously pick my way across the minefield that is socializing and eating out.

All of which is a small price to pay for freedom from pain. I am very happy that I have discovered a road to the future which avoids heavy, chronic medication and repeat prescriptions. These changes to my eating habits have made an amazing difference. It is no exaggeration to say that without them and some carefully chosen vitamin supplements, I would be incapable of walking anywhere and that sitting, standing, or sleeping comfortably would be impossible. I would probably be in a wheelchair, taking several different medications, which would work intermittently. I would probably be knocked out of my head most of the time.

Just to make sure I am not imagining things, I experiment occasionally: I eat a tiny sliver piece of beef, a spoonful or two of rice pudding, or a piece of cheese. More often I forget, tired of the endless calculations behind every meal and end up eating something with tomatoes or red sauce in it for two days in a row. If I am lucky the offending food clears out of my system within twenty-four hours and the pain is lifted.

I don't usually feel that I am missing out, though there are times when I would give anything just to be able to say "Yes, please" to an offer of ice cream, coffee, or cake. Responding "No, thank you" all the time is galling.

It was primarily because of Seline's needs that I was forced to re-evaluate my attitude to pain and driven to experiment. When I looked at the ingredients on baby food, I read closely and began to shop more carefully. It is one of the blessings of having a child, that what I eat has improved tenfold since I became responsible for my daughter's health. Ultimately, I have her to thank for my continued mobility and strength.

Chapter Forty-Six

It is three o'clock in the morning and I should be sleeping. I'm furious with myself, and not because I have been jolted awake by the dulcet tones of my husband's snoring. I woke because I have a head cold, which makes breathing difficult and gives me a headache. But I woke thinking, *what could I do with my impossible hair?* I desperately need a haircut. The answer came to me while I was sleeping that in the meantime, I might wear a headscarf. Without thinking, my inner nag immediately dismissed the idea as ridiculous: "I don't want to look like the Queen!"

With a familiar, clenching wretchedness, I immediately realized that my life only resembles cold porridge because I allow it to. Don't bully yourselves, my children. The story of Auntie Fran's life so far is How Not to Live. If you take nothing else from me, perhaps you may at least collect this understanding: when we allow ourselves to listen to the voice of disapproval for most of our lives, if we are careless in this way, we will probably surround ourselves not with brightness, color, freedom, choices, and good friends, but only with bits and pieces, the butt ends of everyone else's cigarettes: they get to light up, inhale, and blow smoke in our direction. We pick fag ends off the pavement and wonder why life is such a drag.

When I get ill, when I cough and sneeze and blow hot and cold, this is a reminder that I am letting myself live a crap life: that I must propel myself outside and take time to relax in the sunshine. I also need to eat, to treat myself to lunch, instead of surveying the remnants of last night's supper from which I might, if only I am diligent enough, fashion for myself a possible plate of soup. Why live on leftovers? I need to eat fresh food. I am not a dog. Actually, if I were a dog, I would probably treat myself better.

Why have I believed that I am worth less? Not worth the joy and pleased expectations that other people take as their birthright? Voices of disapproval tend to shout more loudly than sweet words of love, so they have claimed my attention. Out of bad habit, I have accepted the critical voice in my head and come to believe that the solidity offered by resentment is the only way out of tiredness and passivity that threatened to drown me. I have gone out of my way to find things to feel resentful about, even though most of this drama was running in my own head. Believing that strife and unhappiness were inevitable, I have put up with half-heartedness, sorrow, and frustration. I have run away many times, from bullies, from unloving boyfriends, from piss-poor jobs. Getting away from the critic in my head is altogether more difficult.

What I can use to help me is recognition. At least I now understand what I am doing and I can use my anger to propel myself away from the habits of self-hatred that are taking too long to die. They are so entrenched that I don't even notice them until they pile up in front of me so that I can hardly move: isolation, insomnia, ill temper, bad food, boredom—all familiar signs that I need to make changes.

There is no time like the present, they say. So tomorrow I may buy a silk scarf—what a gorgeous idea—and a new pair of soft leather gloves to shield my hands from a fresh bout of disapproval; one of my thumbs is badly bitten again, and I want it to heal up quickly. I renew a vow I have made many times, to leave my hands in peace.

I didn't go to town, though I did promise myself I would. Instead, I decided to change the sheets on my daughter's bed, do two loads of washing and get them all dried outside. Not quite the shopping heaven I planned, though I have now made an appointment to get my hair cut, so maybe I will also fit in some lunch and the purchase of scarf and gloves . . . I have to start, sometime, to treat myself like a lady.

On the other hand, my careful shoots of optimism sometimes take a battering. Last week my husband and I went to a different supermarket from our usual. As we left, the pavement sloped down and I pitched forward, dropping the bags I was carrying and clonking my head on a trash can. My specs fell off and I broke a glass jar of large green olives, which wept brine over the pavement. I thought, "At least it is not the eggs" before I wept loudly and got to my feet, slowly rescuing bananas and jettisoning shards of glass as people walked past, unsure how to help. Oddly, I could not stop crying: I was probably slightly concussed. New and shaky caution creeps around the edges of my optimism and will, if I am not careful, make me even less ambitious than usual to venture out, which would be a pity. In this life it seems I will walk a tightrope between normal hopes and bruising reality.

Chapter Forty-Seven

Injustice is what we call something when we do not understand its cause. Injustice is when we ask the question "Why?" and there seems to come no answer. "Why?" has been a question that has consumed my existence. Why me?

I have looked feverishly for answers. I have read obsessively, I have asked questions, and railed against God and the entire universe. I have spent years in compulsive analysis of motives, impulses, trying to discover what makes us tick. The same pre-occupation with knowing why forces me to watch an insect crawling or a leaf unfurling.

I am lucky, I realize, because I am beginning to receive answers to my question. An unanswered "Why?" creates a paralyzing sense of injustice, yet now, because I have answers which, for me, make enough sense of the world, I can get a life. I am freer and can inch myself slowly beyond my inner paralysis.

In a very personal way, I dimly perceive that at a level far above daily living I made a choice to come into this life, in this body, at this time, to experience being me here, now. My heart has also begun to accept some belief in karma, the wheel, which is pushed by the cause and effect we choose, in turn because of our free will. I believe that our creator gives us freedom to choose—a rare privilege—and that we have choices; so in our less laudable careers and actions we may accumulate karmic debts. I emphasize, *these lessons are mine* and they work for me *because they help me to move beyond physical and mental paralysis.* My beliefs are my practical keys for escape. That is all.

So, what now? I have started tweaking some of the usual rules and expectations of daily life to suit myself. I say "no" when I don't want to do something, rather than when I am merely unavailable. I let people down; I disappoint their expectations because there is no use pretending that I can meet them anymore. I realize too, that if I am going to be a let-down, I may as well disappoint for reasons that please me and not only because some find my physical constraints difficult to accept.

When I forget to live consciously, I become a "people pleaser"; then feelings of anger and loss re-surface. I can feel myself becoming cross and sad. Similarly, when I notice in the natural preoccupations of others—for their jobs, their sex lives, their fashion statements—that these interests seem to have passed me by, I feel myself withdrawing from ordinary living. It would be very easy to become isolated again. At times like these, it helps to remember that I can give myself love and acceptance. There is still a large payment due on that account. I also remind myself to accept others *as they are.* To accept life *as it is* becomes the single most important key for my happiness.

It is usually assumed that hard work will see you through and for most of us that belief seems to work well enough. For me, the hardest lesson is that there are always going to be some things I simply cannot work to my will, no matter how hard I try. Instead of risking failure or ridicule, I have faked indifference; have risked being called lazy, a bit of a sloppy flop. Unfortunately, distancing myself from activities I enjoy and which I pretend to dislike only pushes me further away from other people: "Hello! Fran! Are you still there?"

The challenge is to get away from this deadlock and accept some gentle discipline for my temperament, which wants either to sit still or to rush madly. Sitting still goes nowhere, and rushing madly leads to failure. These days I aim for a middle, more measured way to inch me forward in small steps which, taken together, can show me just how far I have come. Then, I can look back with pride and reflect, "See what I chose!"

I will never be a ballet dancer but I still like to dance, so I gyrate in the privacy of my kitchen when no one else is here. From the kitchen window I often watch Eddie and Seline playing football and we wave at each other. I may abandon the dishes and join them outside, where I pretend to be referee. I take part and end up laughing so hard that I almost fall over.

I am learning that it is more restful to give myself time, so that I may walk at ease, appreciate the beauties that can be seen all around me, and not have to stagger painfully, trying to beat the clock.

I console myself that none of my usual daily preoccupations is terribly important. What matters is that I try to show love, to myself and to others. In that spirit, the setbacks we each face can become a source of gentle amusement. Since I am not able to seek for happiness in many of the material goals that others use as their springboards to fulfillment, I must look elsewhere. My search in other directions may sometimes lend me the appearance of having little in common with my friends, yet the main thing that unites us all over time is love.

I have spent the last few years building on that first raft of understanding which Seline illuminated for me. My learning gathers pace as insights follow one after another. Each day I am painting lighter patterns, happier patterns. I am learning that:

- Forgiveness of the past is a gift to all, since forgiveness heals all wounds;
- Acceptance of What Is, is the beginning of self-love;
- Laughter heals; and
- Love makes things better.

I realize now that there is nothing I can do to make myself ugly. I can bite my nails to the quick; I can be cruel or sit at home like a useless lump; I can deny myself pleasure, eat rubbish, and get angry; I can ignore, waste, and squander my talents until they wilt, wither, and die from lack of love; I can forget to ask for what I need. I can overlook all my choices, ignore them, belittle them, dismiss them; I can be hard and calculating, ignoring the lessons of my spirit and the quiet, sweet strengths of my soul. I can live with black and white thinking in an ocean of gray fear and dread; I can punish myself, push myself, and hate myself. Yet nothing I do to hurt myself makes any difference to the truth: my soul knows I am beautiful, even when I forget, or try to kid myself that I am the world's worst person. All the difficulties, challenges, and bitterness I have faced and in some measure, overcome, have made me a better, nicer person. I like the person I am now.

Because of the endless goodness, love, and acceptance that my family and friends show me, and which I am now learning to share with others, I am more aware that I can choose to walk a happier pathway. Happiness is what I choose now. I make a point of smiling and laughing when I don't feel like it and I am finally free of the depression that blighted my young adulthood. I find it easier to accept the help of those who ask "Are you all right?" when I crash painfully—yet again—to the ground and am expected to leap up and, with a beaming smile, offer bright reassurances all round. I appreciate the kindness of passing strangers who stop to help.

I still feel aching sadness which sometimes wells up in me out of nowhere so that I can hardly breathe. When I see a beautiful woman walking nonchalantly where she wishes to go, sometimes I wonder what that would feel like and I long to be her, just for a second, so that I might feel unchained, set free from my lumbering heaviness. I have managed to carve out a simple life of my own choosing. This is no small achievement. So when feelings like these return, I recall the importance of release, of not holding on to the hurt or my sense of loss. I am learning that it is better for me, it is more enjoyable, if I relax, laugh, and go with the flow.

Epilogue

If you ask me now, "What is the point of life?" I answer simply: the point is to keep everything as light as possible: light, as in not heavy and light as in bright. Brightness illuminates our inner compass, which cannot lie to us. All we have to do is trust our feelings and follow the path.

Back when I was a child, I am sure I remember knowing this and being puzzled that all around me, the people I loved were forever insisting on a reality that was heaviness and difficulty, like a backpack full of books that no one wants or needs, but which everyone is reluctant to let go.

I looked on until I too, had learned to believe in the hard stuff. Happily for me, I have been able to unlearn most of it. I have, in some measure, gotten myself back to a lighter place. Deep down I have always known that there is nothing to worry about, that life can be a great big smile, if we let it be. After all the tortuous struggles of growing into adulthood and of proving everyone wrong, now I know that a smile, a kiss, an embrace, and a bit of time spared to rest peacefully together are worth all the stress and graft that mankind ever forced upon itself.

I spent many years living with self-imposed neglect. Until I calmed the fears which travelled everywhere with me, my life resembled a shabby kitchen where a single light bulb hung limply from a frayed flex over my head. The units in this space were old and stained, and licks of paint are peeling off the walls. I didn't bother to hang curtains in the window even for the sake of a little warmth or privacy. The whole place felt riddled with damp, though, as I knew I would be moving soon, it didn't matter. Soon never came. My evenings were spent listening to the wireless while insects buzzed around my face. I was usually working at the kitchen sink, standing uncomfortably. I seldom rested in the single armchair that waited for me at the back of the room.

Change, which I now welcome more freely into my life, has calmed my fears. Filled with a new certainty, I feel immense gratitude to have narrowly escaped the hovel of my old, tired beliefs. In living more comfortably with myself at last, I feel as if I have decided to go for a walk in fresh air. Lacing on a pair of sturdy boots, I pull my hair out of its ties and shake it loose; I place a warm jacket over my shoulders, fumbling at the door catch in my hurry to be away. I don't bother pulling the door closed behind me.

It is beautiful outside. It is late at night and moonlight shines as I pick out a hobblish path down the glinting hillside. There is a rivulet off to my left, gurgling under mossy, damp turf. I know this water is running happily down to the wide sea, which I can hear roaring in the distance. Bats flit breathlessly past. Over my head, clouds scud peacefully, like puffs of smoke from God's pipe.

Here I stand alone, surrounded by everything. This, then, is my real living room, the promise held out for me and for all of Life's precious creatures. Life is far bigger and grander than the cramped, empty cottage that I managed to gouge and scrimp out of fear and hollow sorrows. Reality is a vast universe, so vast that most of the time we are blind to it. Young children know that the world is their oyster. My story shows how I forgot that, only to remember it again, when God's love tapped me on the shoulder and whispered, "I have been waiting for you, my dear."

Acknowledgments

I could not have written this book without the support of my husband. Thanks to Eddie for having faith in me, reading an early draft and suggesting many useful changes. I owe a deep debt of gratitude to my agent, Isabel Atherton of Creative Authors, who believes in my work and always offers indispensable advice and encouragement. I will always be indebted to Skyhorse Publishing, especially to Tony Lyons, my editor Marianna Dworak, and Julie Matysik. Sincere thanks to Colin McPherson for the care and time taken over the jacket photographs. Many thanks to Claire Wingfield for her insightful edits of the manuscript, constant encouragement and timely advice. Thanks to James Macdonald for understanding what cannot be explained. And to my longsuffering family, who have tolerated being misrepresented in these pages with remarkable good humor, I can only say how thankful I am to have been with you all on life's journey. Your enthusiasm has sustained me.